Understanding Medical Informatics

How It *Really* Works

Series Editor
Oleg S. Pianykh

Oleg S. Pianykh

Digital Image Quality
in Medicine

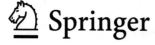 Springer

Oleg S. Pianykh
MGH
Department of Radiology
Harvard Medical School
Newton, MA
USA

ISBN 978-3-319-01759-4   ISBN 978-3-319-01760-0   (eBook)
DOI 10.1007/978-3-319-01760-0
Springer Cham Heidelberg New York Dordrecht London

Printed on acid-free paper

Springer is part of Springer Science+Business Media (www.springer.com)

To my dear wife Dasha,
and our wonderful kids.

Why MI?

Preface 1: The Great Method Gap

Even doctors use it!
Advertisement for popular videoconferencing software

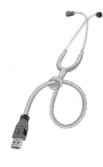

"So, what is medical informatics?" – asked my friend, a bright radiologist, and I suddenly felt that one of us must have dropped from a different planet. Then it had to be me, because my division chair had asked me the same question the day before. After several years and many medical informatics (MI) projects we've done together! Gee, what was going on?

I sat back and took a minute to contemplate my entire career in radiology. The career that started right after earning my computer science and math degrees, when I was looking for the practical beauty to justify the boredom of distilled logic. Was it a wisely chosen path, or had I become a math renegade, a black sheep among white coats?

If you've ever felt lost, welcome to the MI arena. Your medical colleagues, regarding you as something extraterrestrial: "our engineer", "our programmer", or simply "our IT guy". Your math friends, using the word "medical" pejoratively: "How are your rabbits, Fibonacci?"[1] Personally, my academia was the worst: medical journals would hate my formal proofs, while math editors kept crucifying me for the "useless" clinical experiments. As a result, my MI publishing has dwindled to a dragging process of deliberate downgrade, forcing me to remove each half of my work not to appall one half of my audience.

Let's face it: MI brings together two very orthogonal disciplines, medicine and math.[2] Not only do they have very little in common, but their fundamental approaches to reality – experimental in medicine and axiomatic in math – conflict and

---

[1] More on rabbits in http://en.wikipedia.org/wiki/Fibonacci_number

[2] I am putting computer science, statistics, formal logic and a few others under the same math umbrella. In fact, many of my clinical colleagues tend to use the same terminology.

constantly challenge each other. In math, $2+2=4$ regardless of how you do it. In medicine, if two mice out of four died, but the remaining three are still alive, you have to deal with this, period. In math, it is always His Highness Reason who rules and directs His faithful subjects. In medicine, it is always Mother Nature who has the final say. Do they ever listen to each other?

I learned this lesson early, just starting my first hospital job fresh from computer science graduate school. In one of my first meetings I had to explain to my clinical department chair that lossless image compression did not change our images. "It is *lossless,*" – I kept saying, – "It does not change anything by definition!" In the meantime, my respected peer, totally deaf to my exclamations and quietly smiling at my arguments, using his glasses as a magnifier, was meticulously comparing the original and the compressed images side by side and pixel by pixel. With all the patience to ignore me, *he was trying to find the differences between two identical objects.* "The man is downright crazy," I thought, and I'll bet he thought that I was a liar.[3]

Oh, these wonderful stories of applied science – they all sound the same, don't they? The term "*translational* medicine" was well chosen! It was revealing to see the extent to which two different backgrounds made both of us, perfectly sound and rational men, completely incompatible. We spoke different languages. It was truly painful, but it's always been like this. When John Sweeny started one of the first MI departments in the 1980s, he was given the "Doctor of Computer Medicine" title. His colleagues would ask him what it meant. "I treat sick computers" was the answer (Collen 1986).

Has anything changed since then? Computers, statistics, and colorful spreadsheet charts, tossed into this cognitive gap, have made it even wider, turning the slightly questionable into the entirely confusing. We invited the technology to help us, but we hardly spent any time on understanding *how*; we just got too busy with *more important* clinical stuff, you know. But it turned out that reading the table of contents did not amount to reading the entire book; and buying computers and software worked no magic by itself. You simply end up with more computers, more software, less money and (wow!) less patience.[4] So we got upset with the technology we did not bother to comprehend, and our perception of it drifted from inspirational to distractive (Chen et al. 2011). Alas, slowly but surely we've slid into the Great Method Gap: consuming incomprehensible informatics on the clinical side, and multiplying inapplicable applications on the other. Time to get out?

Welcome to this new MI book series, launched with the only goal to bridge the disconnected, and to remove the layers of dusty myths, covering the essence of this most interesting, most current, and most exciting field.

I welcome you, your critique, and your contributions to this series.

Newton, MA, USA   Oleg S. Pianykh

---

[3] Dear Dr. C., if you are reading these lines – you were the best!

[4] This is a perfect illustration of Parkinson's project management law: There is no correlation between the volume of resources assigned to a problem and its importance.

Preface 2: Book Intro

Welcome to the image-is-everything era! Smartphones, tablets, 3D glasses, and even wrist monitors – what's next? Undoubtedly, the list will become obsolete by the time I finish this sentence, but do not blame it on me. Our lives have become image-driven; we *are* pixel addicts.

I had my moment a couple of years ago, aboard a little overcrowded boat that was motoring a bunch of tourists like me to the base of Niagara Falls. As we were approaching this most spectacular point, and as water roared and dense plumes of mist billowed higher and higher, I looked around and saw a quite interesting scene: everyone started reaching for their pockets and bags, pulling out the most diverse arsenal of digital filming technology. By the time we reached the pinnacle of our adventure – the beautiful, massive, mesmerizing waterfall – no one was looking at it! Instead, everybody was filming the thing, taking pictures in front of it, and taking pictures in front of the others taking pictures. "What's wrong with you people," I thought to myself. "You get to experience one of the most fascinating spectacles live, in its full and infinite dimensionality and sound, and you do not care; all you can think about is making cheap snapshots?!" Would you trade the most stunning reality for a pinch of megapixels? And how many megapixels is your reality worth? (Fig. 1)

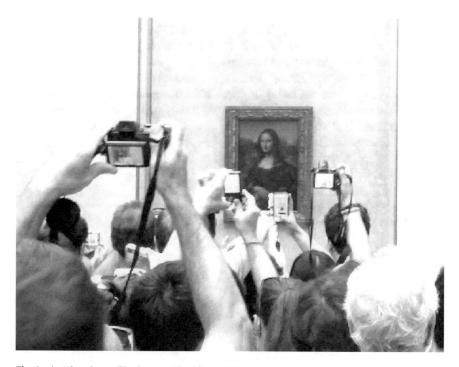

Fig. 1 Another day at The Louvre: "looking at" Giaconda

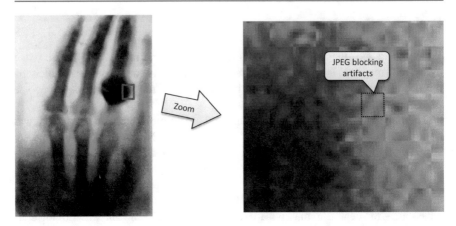

Fig. 2 JPEG compression artifacts (small 8×8 square tiles with abrupt intensity changes on their boundaries)

Then I had another experience, this time while looking for the famous "Frau Roentgen X-ray" online. As you may know, Roentgen's wife was the first inspiration for his imagery – her immortal hand with a wedding ring is now known to many (Fig. 2, left). So I was studying the quality of the early X-rays, and after an hour of web-browsing I found the largest "Frau Roentgen's image" possible. But imagine my disappointment when I discovered that my digital replica was full of lossy compression artifacts (Fig. 2, right). That is, despite the highest resolution and size, the image was absolutely useless, at least for my purposes. Lossy compression had wiped out all of the most intricate features.

And herein lies our first lesson: even the best images can be far from reality, and even the largest images can be far from the best. This matters a lot when we start talking about the diagnostic image value. And it only makes sense to dedicate the first medical informatics book in this series to the diagnostic quality of digital images – before we get lost in our mega-, giga-, and terapixels.

Newton, MA, USA   Oleg S. Pianykh

Reference

Chen, M., Safdar, N., Nagy, P., 2011. Should Medical Schools Incorporate Formal Training in Informatics?. *J. Ditital Imaging*, pp. 1–5.
Collen, M. F., 1986. Origins of medical informatics. *Western Journal of Medicine*, pp. 778–785.

Acknowledgements

To my dear family,

To all my colleagues – for asking questions, and for answering mine,

To Sean Doyle – for his valuable feedback on the compression discussion,

To Vassilios Raptopoulos, M.D., Alexander Bankier, M.D., Diana Litmanovich, M.D., Melvin Clouse, M.D. – for many years of interesting projects.

To you, my dear reader, for taking the time. Whatever you think of this book, please let me know; your praise and your rotten tomatoes can reach me at opiany@gmail.com.

Contents

A Bit of History and Touch of Philosophy

I think, therefore I am
Descartes, *Principles of Philosophy*
I am. I am, I exist, I think, therefore I am; I am
because I think, why do I think? I don't want to think
anymore, I am because I think that I don't want to
be, I think that I … because … ugh!

Jean-Paul Sartre, *Nausea*

When I was a math student, I was positively certain that all "history of mathematics" books were written by losers incapable of making real math breakthroughs. I was young and ignorant back then, but at least one of these vices was cured by time.

Then recently I was asked to teach MI to math students, and I realized how many things I've taken for granted, without even thinking about their meaning and roots. Teaching MI to a medical audience is easy: anything "medical" puts them at ease right away. But once you go outside this box, you'll be surprised, and you'll be challenged.

Anticipating this challenge before beginning with my new audience, I sat down and tried to understand—for the first time—the origins of MI. It was worth the time. The "early MI" stories, covered with the patina of folklore, proved to be incredibly captivating. The most open-minded historians traced MI back to the first punch-cards, automobiles, telegraph, telephone, radio—virtually any technology that advanced human productivity (Fig. 1.1). Looking at this bottomless history, at some point I thought that I shouldn't be surprised to discover that Ramses or Alexander the Great ran their own MI shops; just like "computers" used to be human, "tablets" used to be clay (Birchette 1973). Ironically, my suspicion turned out to be right: the real Imhotep (twenty-seventh century BC), despite his distorted pop-culture image, was known as the earliest physician *and* engineer (Anon. n.d.).

In short, MI proved to be a fairly ancient science, but its aging wrought a peculiar problem. Somehow, as the time was flying by, it became increasingly fashionable to define MI through this popular technology. That is, the ubiquitous technology used *anywhere else*. All of a sudden, radios and punch-cards started to take over, eclipsing something je-ne-sais-quoi, very subtle yet fundamentally imperative.

So what have we fallen into missing? Ledley's work (Ledley and Lusted 1959) is definitely the best place to start looking for answers. Published in 1959—the era when "computer" meant a set of wooden pegs to sort punch-cards —the paper introduced an entirely different MI definition: it's not about the tools, it's about thinking. Being a physician, Ledley observed that our clinical reasoning can be translated into

O.S. Pianykh, *Digital Image Quality in Medicine*, Understanding Medical Informatics,
DOI 10.1007/978-3-319-01760-0_1, © Springer International Publishing Switzerland 2014

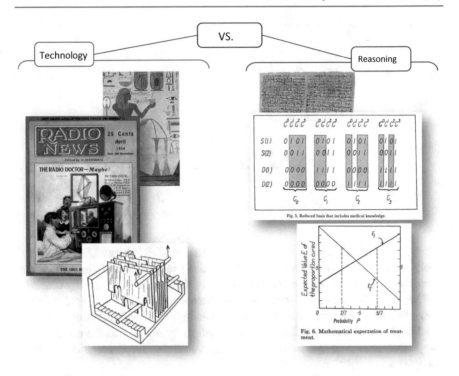

Fig. 1.1 Early origins of MI: technology (radio, punch cards) vs, reasoning (Edwin Smith papyrus attributed to Imhotep, Ledley's mathematical reasoning in medicine)

formal logical terms; *diagnostic reasoning is mathematical.*[1] And if that is the case, math and technology integrate naturally with clinical work *provided that* they fit the intrinsic logic of your analysis. Without this umbilical cord, playing with cool techy gadgets becomes pointless.

I think this was the most essential statement about MI from which to begin. And that's how it started to evolve: in the 1960s, we had the first MI publications and research groups, although the term "medical informatics" wasn't coined until the 1970s. The 1970s also saw the advent of computed tomography—the first purely computed medical imaging, a true success of bringing the physicians and the engineers together. In the 1980s, we had 50 professional MI societies. I recommend Collen (1986) as another historically interesting reference: penned midway between Ledley's and our times, it gives an interesting perspective on the early MI developments now all but forgotten.

---

[1] This connects us to the Church-Turing principle, which in its essence states that computing devices reflect the way humans think and process data—the fundamental assumption that started the whole field of computer science. This is exactly what we observe with contemporary decision support in medicine.

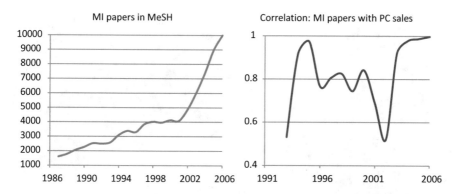

Fig. 1.2 MI literature trends. *Left*: MI papers in Medical Subject Headings (MeSH), identified by (Deshazo et al. 2009); note explosive growth after the year 2000. *Right*: Correlating MI MeSH papers with global computer sales, on a 4-year basis (from each year to 4 years back). Note how near to perfect the correlation has been in recent years. Are MI publications driven by sheer computer sales?

In short, things moved quickly but predictably until the late 1980s saw a swift disruption in the alluring romance of old science and new technology. The computer genie was unleashed, rapidly flooding medicine with all the tools it could ever dream of. In a couple of short decades the field of medicine went through the full swing of IT revolution, digital standardization, and skyrocketing counts of MI publications (Deshazo et al. 2009) (Fig. 1.2). Physicians who started their careers with film and stethoscopes were buried under an avalanche of techy offers that they really did not have the time and the skills to follow. The faster-evolving technology started to spin away from the medical thinking, and we started to lose the early MI "reasoning defines methodology" principle. We started calling MI anything with an "OK" button.

This led to a rather ironic situation, when 50 years after Ledley's mind-bridging work, Schuemie and colleagues (Schuemie et al. 2009) had to define MI *recursively*—that is, by taking the volume of all MI-labeled publications, and trying to keyword-cluster them just to find out what their authors meant by "medical informatics" (Fig. 1.3). Undoubtedly, this exercise in existentialism[2] was very instructive in defining the current MI frontiers. But it was equally instructive in proving that any science should be defined and driven by its core meaning, and not by an overdosage of its referencing.

We have entered the era when informational technology has become a commodity, and bringing iPads to hospitals – a great MI project. Seasoned with a head-spinning rush of IT upgrades and updates, monthly gadget releases and gibberish IT trends, this produced a fast-tech diet upsetting canonical medical minds. "I die of thirst beside the fountain[3]": we could not handle it anymore. So we stopped, and we felt the strange urge to go back to our good old stethoscopes, so consistent and so trusty.

---

[2] "You are – your life, and nothing else," as Sartre once suggested.

[3] Borrowing from my favorite François Villon.

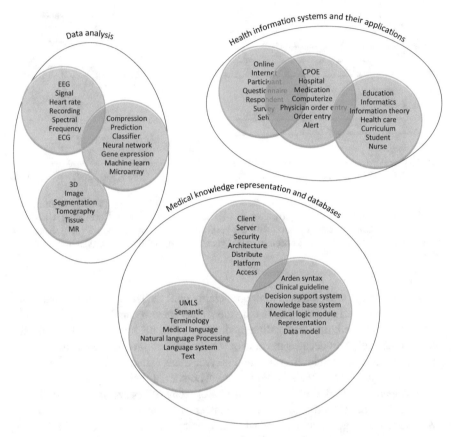

Fig. 1.3   Schuemie and colleagues clustered 3,660 articles from 16 MI journals, published in 2005–2008, to find out what their authors meant by "medical informatics"

▶ *Nota bene:* It is surprising to see how many MI classes at our medical schools are reduced to the "web browsing for doctors"-like trivia. If we think that this is what MI is about, we've got a serious problem already. Besides, let's not forget that modern medical students have been web-browsing since their kindergarten years, and they certainly do not need to be lectured on this while getting their MD degrees.

I remember how some 15 years ago I was teaching one of my elderly clinical colleagues to double-click, but we did not call it "medical informatics"…

So I offer you a little challenge, my dear colleagues: take the original cartesian premise of Ledley's thought-driven MI, and try to map it onto the current state of our miserable art, which I have sketched in Fig. 1.4. Doesn't really fit, does it? From the current point of view, Imhotep, Asclepius, Hippocrates, or Leonardo were true job-hackers: they looked for the shortest path from the problem to the solution,

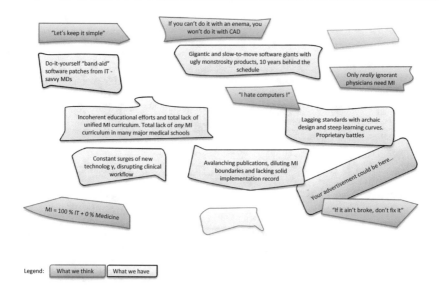

Fig. 1.4 Building blocks and decision paradigms of current MI – ready for your projects?

inventing the technology accordingly. These days, we often start from technology, acting as if chicken soup came before the chicken and the egg. But you cannot buy a lavishly-expensive IT product, shove it down the throats of your doctors, and call it a great technology triumph. It is nothing but a disaster, and it should be avoided at any cost.

One of my longtime friends kept saying that he enjoys reading science papers from the 1970s much more than the current stuff. "They did not have the computers back then", – he'd say – "So they had to think". He was young and very far from being a backward-looking conservative, and he made a good historical point. In my own case, it was not until I read those old papers that I realized what MI is about.

References

Anon., n.d. Edwin Smith Papyrus. [Online] Available at: http://en.wikipedia.org/wiki/Edwin_Smith_papyrus [Accessed 01 May 2013].

Birchette, K. P., 1973. The history of medical libraries from 2000 B.C. to 1900 A.D.. Bull Med Libr Assoc, pp. 302–308.

Collen, M. F., 1986. Origins of medical informatics. West J Med, pp. 778–785.

Deshazo, J. P., Lavallie, D. L. & Wolf, F. M., 2009. Publication trends in the medical informatics literature: 20 years of "Medical Informatics" in MeSH. BMC Med Inform Decis Mak.

Ledley, R. S. & Lusted, L. B., 1959. Reasoning Foundations of Medical Diagnostics. Science, 3 July. pp. 9–21.

Schuemie, M. J., Talmon, J. L., Moorman, P. W. & Kors, J. A., 2009. Mapping the domain of medical informatics. Methods Inf Med, pp. 76–83.

Part I

Do No Harm

Digital Images and Digital Myths

Let's begin with a short quiz.

Which of the following digital image transforms can be done *without* losing the original image quality?

– Digital image zoom
– Digital image rotation

Don't rush, and think about this for a moment. Obviously, these two are the most essential image transformations. They give us the ability to handle digital images in the same way the pros from a bygone era used to work with old films—turning them around or looking at them through a magnifying glass. Clearly, the films were not altered. But what about the "soft copies"?

You might be surprised but both transforms, when applied to the digital images, will *worsen* their quality. The quality drop may not be visible, but this surely doesn't mean that it doesn't exist. Moreover, it's cumulative: the more digital zooming and rotation you apply, the worse the images become (Fig. 2.1). Why?

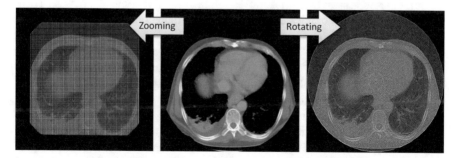

Fig. 2.1 Visualizing interpolation errors. The image in the *center* is the original; the image on the *left* is the result of 20 cumulative zooms by 20 % (in and out); the image on the *right* is the result of 20 cumulative rotations by 16 degrees (counter- and clockwise). In theory, *left* and *right* images should be identical to the original, as each transform was repeated to cancel itself. In reality however, each zoom or rotation has added invisible errors, accumulated into impossible-to-ignore distortion

O.S. Pianykh, *Digital Image Quality in Medicine*, Understanding Medical Informatics,   9
DOI 10.1007/978-3-319-01760-0_2, © Springer International Publishing Switzerland 2014

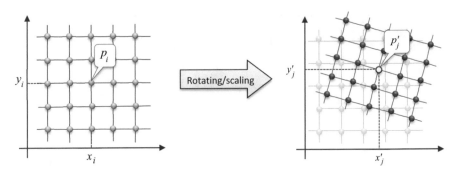

Fig. 2.2 Original digital image is a matrix of integer pixel values (*green dots*), sampled at specific discrete locations (x_i,y_i). When this image is rotated or zoomed, we need to know the new pixel values p_j', corresponding to the new locations (x_j',y_j') (*red dots*). The new points (x_j',y_j') are not present in the original, so the only way to approximate their p_j' values is to use interpolation from the known grid values

The problem lies in the very nature of digital images. Unlike its analog film predecessor, a digital image is a very rigid structure; stored as a $W \times H$ matrix of integer[1] pixel values p_i, measured (sampled) at integer pixel locations (x_i,y_i): $x_i = 1,\dots,W$ (image width), and $y_i = 1,\dots,H$ (image height), as shown in Fig. 2.2. This grid of $W \times H$ integers p_i is really all this digital image knows about the original, real object.

But when you zoom or rotate, you will need to know the pixel values p_j' at some new locations x_j', y_j' that fall between the lines of the existing grid (Fig. 2.2, right). Where can you get those new values, you ask? Nowhere: the image has already been taken, and it simply does not contain any measurements other than the original p_i at the original (x_i,y_i) grid. So your only recourse is to *approximate* p_j' from the known p_i around it.

For instance, if (x_j',y_j') = (10.123, 87.916), you can say that it is "close enough" to the known integer (x_i,y_i) = (10,88), and use p_i at this location as an approximation to p_j' at (10.123, 87.916). This is called "nearest neighbor" approximation (interpolation), the roughest and most primitive approach to "inventing" the new p_j. There are many other more complex and far cleverer interpolation techniques; see a great review by Lehmann and colleagues (Lehmann et al. 1999). However, none of them can solve the fundamental "missing data" problem, since any approximation of the *unknown* cannot be exact; "close enough" is not the same as "exactly equal". Hence the distortions and inevitable loss of quality in any zoomed or rotated image.

And the quality distortion story continues ad infinitum, repeating itself with virtually any digital image transform: changing intensities, performing lossy compression, using image registration, applying image filters, and so forth. Replacing the original image with a modified one nearly always means some loss of the original image information. Take image filters, for instance: many of us must have heard

---

[1] Some more advanced image formats do support decimal (float-precision) pixels. But they are rare, and they must use finite-precision computer math anyway.

about denoising filtering, removing pixel noise (such as low-dose noise in CT) to make diagnostically-important details more visible. I have seen a number of radiologists asking the same obvious question: If a single pass of a denoising filter makes an image better, why can't we apply it 10 or 100 times, and get the most improved picture? Well, because it is very much like drinking good old wine from your vineyard[2]: one glass can make you better, but knock back 10 or 100..., and that's a whole different story. In the same way, any digital transform has its own "distortion toll", and it is cumulative: when you do too many, it can get extremely ugly.

Therefore, making a good diagnostic CT or MR scan is only the beginning. Keeping it good and diagnostically-sound is a much more difficult proposition, often neglected or forgotten. With anything digital, the assumption of persistent original quality paves the straight road to hell. The rest of this book is dedicated to learning better options.

▶ *Nota bene:* The only way to counteract the negative effects of image transformations is to always keep a copy of the original image. For instance, when you are zooming into an image on a PACS workstation, PACS software should be smart enough to keep track of the cumulative zoom factor. Then this single zoom can be applied to the original image, instead of progressively zooming already distorted results of the previous zooms. This single-zoom approach is indeed already programmed into most applications, but some memory-limited ones (such as those running images on smartphones or embedded systems) may choose to drop the original image to free up the limited memory. In this case, the distortions will inevitably become cumulative.

Reference

Lehmann, T. M., Gönner, C., Spitzer, K., 1999. "Survey: interpolation methods in medical image processing", *IEEE Trans Med Imaging*, pp. 1049–1075.

---

[2] If you are in medicine, I suppose you have one? What, not even a wine cellar? OK, OK, a bottle of Bud at your friend's party :)

Image Interpolation

3

Key Points

Image interpolation is required to approximate image pixels at the locations where they were not known originally. As a result, any imaging software will be applying interpolation on a regular basis. Replacing the original image with interpolated will result in visible image distortion, artifacts, and the loss of diagnostic image quality. The proper choice of the interpolation algorithm can keep these distortions at minimum.

Digital interpolation is one of the best-kept secrets in medical imaging. Everyone has "kind of" heard about it, but only a few know what it really does. Nonetheless, its effects on diagnostic image quality are profound, and must not be ignored.

As previously mentioned, interpolation computes pixel values at the locations where they were not originally defined (Fig. 2.2). Even the most trivial digital transforms such as zoom or rotation will displace pixel dots from their original grid, and therefore will require interpolation.[1] This makes interpolation indispensable, which is why it's so ubiquitous, although you may be unaware of it. Moreover, it is used on the most impressive scale. As an example, consider a typical MR image, acquired with the standard $W \times H = 256 \times 256$ resolution; and consider yourself, looking at this image full-screen on a rather modest $1{,}024 \times 1{,}024$ display. Quite a mundane setup, but even here, the original image has already been forsaken. What you're looking at has been resized to the new $W' \times H' = 1{,}024 \times 1{,}024$ resolution. That's 4 times the original along each image dimension, thus containing 16 times more pixels. Where did all these new pixels come from? Clearly, they are introduced by the interpolation algorithm, which added 15 new pixels for each original one. Put another way, in that full-screen $1{,}024 \times 1{,}024$ MR image you are looking at, at most $1/16 = 6\%$ of all pixels can be original. The other 94 % *are entirely simulated by the interpolation routine*. Quite an impressive image modification indeed, wouldn't you say?

---

[1] Examples of less-trivial image transformations include nonlinear image registration, 3D rendering, functional maps, etc.

O.S. Pianykh, *Digital Image Quality in Medicine*, Understanding Medical Informatics, 13
DOI 10.1007/978-3-319-01760-0_3, © Springer International Publishing Switzerland 2014

This fact alone should make you exceptionally cautious about the choice and performance of the interpolating algorithm; there are plenty of possible interpolation techniques that use different logic to balance performance versus quality. But what makes it really significant is the naïve persistence with which we keep inviting more and more interpolation, without even thinking about it. The most popular image quality myth, universally repeated by vendors and echoed by their overly-devoted users is "The higher the monitor resolution, the better the image". I hope that by now you see where the "myth" part is coming from: the more display resolution exceeds the original images dimensions, the more interpolation will be needed to rescale the image, and the less original data you will see. Adding more water to your tea does not make more tea; but it sure turns your tea into water.

So let's delve a little deeper into the process of interpolation, to understand its tradeoffs.

3.1   How Does Interpolation Work?

Figure 3.1 shows the basics of digital interpolation. For simplicity, we use a one-dimensional example (applicable to interpolating audio or ECG), but two-dimensional image interpolation is most frequently performed as a combination of two one-dimensional interpolations along image x and y axes[2] (Fig. 3.1, right).

In this example, to approximate pixel value p_x at the unknown location x, the interpolation algorithm will attempt to "restore" the missing continuous data by fitting a continuous curve into the known (original) discrete samples $p_i = \{p_1, p_2, p_3, p_4\}$. The choice of the fitting technique defines the choice of the interpolation algorithm. For example, we can consider the simplest continuous fit – a straight line – passing through p_2 and p_3, the two closest neighbors of the unknown p_x. The equation for this

line is $p_x^L(x) = \dfrac{p_2(x_3 - x) + p_3(x - x_2)}{x_3 - x_2}$, and this is how we determine the

interpolated value of p_x^L at any x. You can easily verify that $p_x^L(x_2) = p_2$ and $p_x^L(x_3) = p_3$, meaning that the linear interpolation is exact for the two known pixels p_2 and p_3; so you can expect it to perform "reasonably well" at some arbitrary x between x_2 and x_3 – *assuming* that the intensity change follows a linear pattern.

Yet other assumptions can lead to other interpolating rules. For example, we could say that to make our interpolation more accurate, we have to use two neighbors on each side, thus fitting a smooth curve through all four $p_i = \{p_1, p_2, p_3, p_4\}$. This leads to a *higher-order* cubic interpolation, with p_x^C being a cubic interpolation result for p_x (Fig. 3.1). As you can see, the linearly-interpolated p_x^L differs from the cubic-interpolated p_x^C. That is, different interpolation algorithms produce different interpolation results. But this is inevitable: we used different assumptions for each of these techniques. Furthermore, since the true p_x is unknown, all our assumptions remain entirely hypothetical.

---

[2] This is why you can find the "bi" prefix in the image interpolation algorithm names: "bilinear", "bicubic".

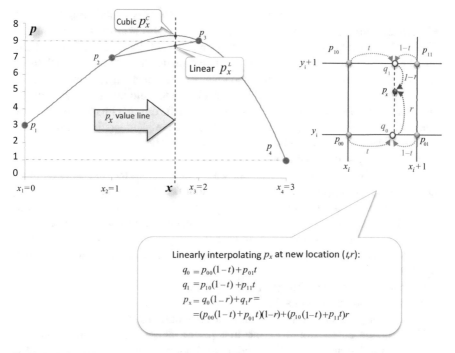

Fig. 3.1 *Left*: Interpolating unknown pixel value p_x at its new location x, using different interpolation approaches. *Right*: Using two 1D linear interpolations in 2D, to interpolate unknown p_x from its four neighbors p_{00}, p_{10}, p_{01}, p_{11}. First, linear interpolation is used in the horizontal direction to compute points q_0 and q_1; then it's applied vertically to compute p_x from q_0 and q_1

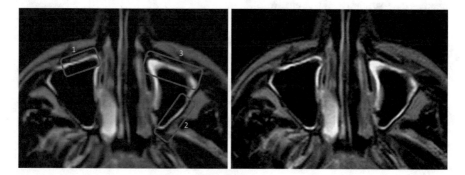

Fig. 3.2 Same image opened in two different PACS (Picture Archiving and Communication System) apps. Note severe aliasing artifacts ("staircasing", blur) on the left image, displayed with an inferior interpolation algorithm (Pianykh 2012)

Therefore let's make a brief mental stop here, and take our first learning point: one can suggest diverse interpolation algorithms, which will produce equally diverse outcomes. In practical terms, this means that the same image displayed in different imaging software can appear strikingly different. Look at Fig. 3.2 – it shows *the same* MR image, opened in *two different* medical imaging applications. Both claim diagnostic image quality, but the one on the left clearly uses a more primitive interpolation technique, most likely linear, leading to very visible artifacts (can you spot them in the selected areas?). The program on the right, by contrast, runs a more intricate interpolation algorithm, such as cubic or better. The "broken lines" disappear in areas 1 and 2, details and boundaries become much sharper in area 3. It's easy to run into cases where primitive interpolation techniques could significantly undermine the diagnostic image quality, even when the original image is perfect and intact. Conclusion: checking for proper interpolation implementation must become an imperative item on your clinical software shopping list.

How would you do this check?

Theoretically, you could ask your software vendor about the interpolation algorithm they are using, and watch the wide range of facial expressions corresponding to the "Why are you torturing me with this nonsense?" state of mind. Besides, as we've mentioned so many times, it is really all about fitting your image data with the best choice of the interpolation algorithm. So take the ultimate medical informatics approach of "theory meets practice" and work similarly to what is shown in Fig. 3.2:

– Open a relatively small image that has sharp edges
– Zoom into the edges with at least a factor of 3
– Look for any unusual artifacts around the edge outlines

Sharp image edges would be the first places where simplistic interpolations would fail, producing jaggies, blur, and other abnormal pseudo-details. Other good candidates include thin structures (small vessels, fractures, etc.), small objects (nodules, bifurcations), objects of known shapes (circular or linear). Check them as well, especially if they matter in your work. Finally, try to open the same images in another program; cross-software, cross-vendor comparison is often the best way to answer the "What's going on?" question.

▶ *Nota bene:* Medical imaging software vendors (and I have been in these shoes myself, running a PACS startup) would know one of the most frequent user complaints: "The images in your program look terrible!" This may sound strange to an unprepared ear – why would the same image look different in a different program? But it is real as we have just seen, and it echoes the same interpolation phenomena, subconsciously upsetting a trained clinical eye. Having a good original image is not enough. Displaying it with a good interpolation technique is the key.

3.2   Interpolation Artifacts

We've already touched on the subject of interpolation artifacts, but let's give it a bit more thought. What is an interpolation artifact anyway?

The answer to this question is far from being trivial: the entire interpolation, as we know, is one big artifact – an artificial attempt to miraculously generate pixel data at locations where it's never been collected. Sometimes it may work well, but sometimes it may produce highly abnormal patterns, which could not exist in the original however it was acquired. Therefore we can define interpolation artifacts as extremely unnatural and visible deviations, impossible with the original data.

Figure 3.3 shows a fragment from the image Fig. 3.2, zoomed with a 15x factor by four different interpolation algorithms. If we do not use any continuous fitting at all, and simply enlarge every original image pixel, we end up with image A – a pretty dull "staircasing", where each single point constitutes the most unnatural artifact.[3] If we use linear interpolation (image B), the outcome is discernibly better: most of the pixel boundaries are smoothed away by the now-linear gradients. However, the flip side of this smoothing is blur or visible loss of sharpness, which is another well-known interpolation problem, the opposite of staircasing. In addition, the assumption of linear intensity gradients (the fundamental assumption of the linear interpolation) fails on the sharp, nonlinear image boundaries and clearly suffers from the same "staircasing" artifact (area B1 in Fig. 3.3).

Cubic interpolation (image C in Fig. 3.3) does a bit better job, further reducing staircasing in some areas (such as C1 and C2, improved compared to image B). In fact, using cubic with less demanding zooms of up to 4x might be sufficient to make a decent image, which is why this algorithm has been so popular in diagnostic imaging software. Nevertheless, cubic interpolation comes with its own peculiarities. One of them can be seen in Fig. 3.1: doesn't it bother you that the value of $p_x{}^C$ turned out to be *larger* than any of the original pixel values $p_i = \{p_1, p_2, p_3, p_4\}$ around it?

Practically this means that pixel $p_x{}^C$, inserted by the cubic interpolation into the modified image, will look brighter than any of its neighbors. This is exactly what happened in the C2 area of image C (Fig. 3.3), shown as a contrast-enhanced inlay C3. Note the unusually-bright blob in the middle of it. Known as a "ringing artifact", it comes from local peaks in the nonlinear interpolating functions.[4] The original data (image A) has absolutely no bright spots in this location.

Well, this is exactly the point where you start feeling the bias of *any* interpolation technique, regardless of its design and complexity. And this is the bias which will keep interfering with your diagnostic interpretations. The bright blob in C3 makes perfect sense in terms of cubic interpolation, curving up around the $p_x{}^C$ point, but it certainly may not make any sense in terms of the original data. For example, it may so happen that the highest original brightness p_3 (Fig. 3.1) already contains the maximum possible pixel value for this particular image, and going anywhere above that value would simply be illegal. Or chances are that all $p_i = \{p_1, p_2, p_3, p_4\}$ belong to a particular tissue type, and $p_x{}^C$, jumping above them with significantly different color, will be misidentified as diagnostic abnormality or pathology. But – remember? – $p_x{}^C$ is *not* a part of the original data (!), and although you see it on the screen in your zoomed or rotated image, you cannot make any diagnostic decisions based on its value. Pretty hard, when the absolute majority of the pixels you see are non-original, isn't it?

---

[3] Note that our definition of "natural" is based entirely on our subjective expectations for normal human imaging and anatomy. The same "staircasing" interpolation would have worked perfectly for a chessboard image.

[4] Linear interpolation, as a linear function, cannot have local peaks.

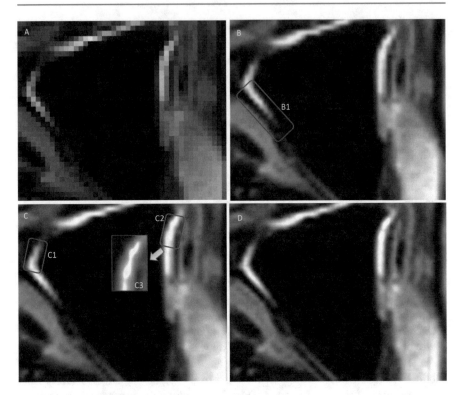

Fig. 3.3 Different interpolation algorithms at work at 15x image zoom: *A* – plain "nearest neighbor" zooming without continuous interpolation (turning original pixels into large tiles with constant intensity); *B* – linear interpolation; *C* – cubic interpolation, *D* – L2-optimal interpolation developed in (Pianykh 2012). Example *A* is the only option preserving the original pixel values, but its quality is clearly inadequate for any practical use. Linear interpolation *B* does much better, but with visible blur. Cubic in *C* improves the contrast (lost in *B*), but may have ringing artifacts (abnormally-bright spots in the selected area), and still suffers from "staircasing" on the sharp boundaries. *D* solves most of the interpolation problems (The differences between these images are more obvious when seen on monitors rather when viewed in print)

Interpolation artifacts reflect the essence of any mathematical modeling: whatever you assume in the model will appear in the final results. Even the most sophisticated math cannot resurrect the dead-missing original data. This should make you more cautious, especially with significant interpolation use such as high-factor zooms.

As you should realize by now, blur, staircasing, and "ringing" (with bright or dark spots) are the first indications of an insufficient or failing interpolation routine. So when you suspect an interpolation artifact, use the simple trick we suggested earlier. Zoom your image a bit in and out, and see what happens to that suspicious area. If it keeps the same appearance, shape, size, and relative position, then most likely it was part of the original data. But if it starts moving with respect to its neighbors, or changes its brightness and visual pattern – then you can be sure you have an "interpolation imposter". Interpolation artifacts are largely affected by current interpolation settings, such as zoom ratio.

▶ *Nota bene:* As mentioned earlier, interpolation artifacts can be found in virtually all areas of medical imaging. Partial volume artifacts, abundant in 3D CT scans, are largely due to inter-voxel interpolation. The same can be said about the lowered resolution in perfusion maps, where interpolation is used both in spatial and temporal domains (Pianykh 2012). Since any digital data is acquired in discrete samples, interpolation is the only way to keep filling in the blanks, and artifacts cannot be avoided. But they surely can be managed with the appropriate choice of interpolation algorithm.

3.3 Interpolation Roundoffs

Asking really dumb questions is… the most important part of any understanding. When my students start with a "Sorry, I have a really stupid question" introduction, I know that something interesting is coming. So I'd like to ask you one of these questions: what is the average of 2 and 3?

Did you say 2.5? Are you really, really sure?

The correct answer is "it depends", as strange as that may sound. But it's true, because it depends on your *data format*. If you tell me that you drink 2.5 cups of coffee per day on average, it certainly does not mean that you have a half-broken cup, which you enjoy after the first two. Well, the same is true of images, and of computers in general: they store data up to a specific precision. And in the case of pixels, it is virtually always the "zero decimals", integer precision – image pixels are stored as integer numbers.[5]

This simple fact greatly affects all image manipulations, interpolation included. If you need to interpolate the unknown pixel p_x half-way between the original pixels with values 2 and 3, using simple linear interpolation, you will find that $p_x^L = 2.5$, but you cannot store 2.5 in an integer pixel value. Therefore, you need to round it off to the nearest integer such as 3 in our example. And voilà, the average of 2 and 3 becomes 3. This roundoff is required to preserve the integer pixel format, but you do lose the fractional part. And "losing" means introducing new errors into your diagnostic data (Fig. 3.4).

Once introduced, these errors never do go away; after multiple interpolations, they only accumulate and grow larger. This is another reason why repetitive digital image manipulations lead to extremely ugly results, as we saw in Fig. 2.1. So it's not only the interpolation artifacts, but the roundoffs as well, that destroy the original image quality. In addition to this, roundoffs are responsible for steamrolling fine image details or even moving some of them around.

We illustrate roundoff problems in more detail in Fig. 3.5, which considers three neighboring pixel values of 1, 2 and 3, taken from a single pixel line in the original image. Imagine that the image has to be zoomed in (resized) at 3x factor – then you

---

[5] For example, DICOM would use 16 bits per pixel to store grayscale medical images, such as X-rays, MRI or CT.

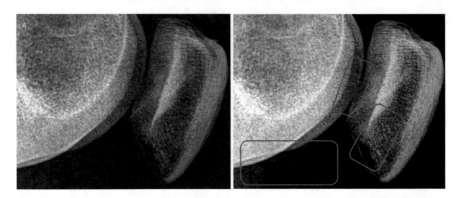

Fig. 3.4 Pure roundoff errors (with no interpolation involved). Image (**A**) shows the original, and (**B**) rounding pixel values to multiples of 20. You can see how image details disappear and shading becomes much flatter (compare the selected areas to the original)

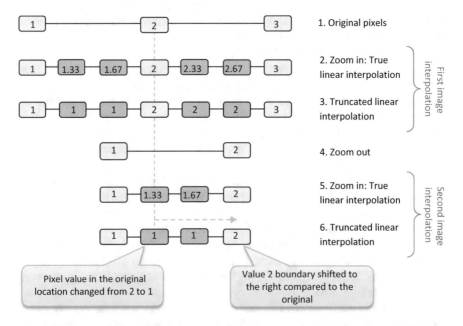

Fig. 3.5 Two rounds of interpolation with integer truncation, and their effects on the image pixels, taken from a single pixel line. As you can see, even pixel values at the original locations can change due to cumulative truncation artifacts

have to insert two interpolated pixels between any two original ones. Then linear continuous interpolation kicks in at step 2, but produces non-integer values in the interpolated locations. Therefore the non-integers will be truncated at step 3, and these will be the pixels you will see in the interpolated image.

Now this resized image can be zoomed out to its original size. This will drop most of the intermediate pixels. However, interpolation has no "memory" of the original vs. inserted data, so it may drop the original pixels and keep the interpolated only, just like pixels 1 and 2 at step 4. If you have to zoom again later, you will have to repeat the truncated interpolation at steps 5 and 6, degrading the original quality even further. So it comes as no surprise that even the original pixel locations (such as pixel 2 in the first line) can lose their true values. And if value 2 corresponded to a particular organ or structure boundary important to us, we would see it shift to the right from its original location. Truncated interpolation will *dislocate* the original image details.

▶ *Nota bene:* One of my colleagues was involved in clinical data analysis, that required very accurate – pixel to pixel – image registration (positioning). All of a sudden she discovered that some of her images did not match: they appeared shifted by one pixel along the main image diagonal. It turned out that some images had gone through truncated interpolation after acquisition. Truncation had introduced the shifts.

In this way, and with only two resizing steps, we managed to inflict sufficient damage on the original data, and integer truncation was mainly responsible for that. When the interpolation is done for display purposes only, and the original image data has still been preserved, you can always return to the original. However, if you start resizing the images, saving modified copies, and, even worse, resizing those copies again, beware! You can lose the original diagnostic information faster than you can imagine.

3.4   Interpolation and Performance

"OK, OK, there are better and worse interpolation techniques; I get it," you might be saying, "But why don't you people just agree on the best ones and use them all the time?" If MDs can follow the "best practices" logic, why can't you?

We'd love to, had we had the resources.

Let's take our "cubic vs. linear" example from Fig. 3.1. Cubic interpolation is more powerful, but it processes more input data (four points $\{p_1, p_2, p_3, p_4\}$ instead of two $\{p_2, p_3\}$ for the linear), and computes a more complex formula (see Sect. 3.5). This penalizes performance, making cubic interpolation several times slower than linear. If you run it on a big fat workstation, zooming into a reasonably small image, you won't have a problem. But when you need it on a simple laptop (not to mention, smartphone), for large image data; when you need it interactively, the performance toll can become heavy and very noticeable. Your program will start "freezing", and given the fact that interpolation is used all the time, this will drive you crazy in no time flat.

▶ *Nota bene:* Another reason for linear interpolation popularity lies in the fact that it is natively supported by all graphics programming interfaces, used by imaging software developers: OpenGL, DirectX, CUDA, Windows API functions, and others. That is, software developers do not have to write any linear interpolation code – it is built in. But for cubic and even more advanced interpolation types, this is not the case; they do require coding and a good knowledge of interpolation fundamentals. Unfortunately, not too many developers would have the time and inclination to roll up their sleeves for that.

We can certainly hope that computing power will continue to grow, but so does image volume, and the most powerful CPU will sooner or later find some overwhelming data that it cannot process in real-time. Image interpolation, on the contrary, has to be real-time all the time. Therefore software developers must balance quality against performance, in order to keep their often impatient customers happy. One simple trick used all the time is switching between the simple (fast) and quality (slow) interpolation routines depending on the user input. Figure 3.6 illustrates this approach.

In most clinical software, images can be zoomed interactively, by dragging a mouse over them. While dragging, you may see some deterioration in the zoomed image quality; to support interactive zooms, the software must run a simple and fast interpolation algorithm (Fig. 3.6, left). But once you stop zooming (by releasing the mouse button, for instance), the image will redraw with much better quality – this is exactly when quality (slower) interpolation kicks in (Fig. 3.6, right). In this way, the slower interpolation is used only once at the end of your zooming selection, which makes its processing time unperceivable, and its final result – perfect. Faster interpolation, on the other hand, is used only to support your intermediate interactive zooming, but does not affect the final image appearance.

Performance cost is also the reason why some applications do not support interactive interpolations at all. In most cases, instead of continuous interactive zooming they offer only discrete incremental zooms – by a factor of 2, for instance. In this case, the number of interpolations is reduced to one per zooming step, and this can be done in real time as well. This approach is most common on devices with relatively slow CPUs, such as mobile tablets and smartphones.

Finally, performance is often the reason for using interpolation where it was not even needed – that is, when pixel locations and values remain intact. Consider any time-consuming image processing such as perfusion analysis of temporal CT and MR series. To compute perfusion values (maps), one needs to solve complex perfusion equations at *each* pixel, which becomes very time-consuming. This is why perfusion software implementations prefer to compute the true values on a reduced pixel grid (skipping every second or third pixel, for instance), then interpolating the values for the skipped pixels. Even skipping every other pixel in x and y direction gives us a 4x performance improvement – a very substantial speedup assuming we can leave with some possible interpolation artifacts (Fig. 3.7). 3D image rendering, and other complex processing routines will rely heavily on this same approach.

To conclude – interpolation is a great tool, but as with any other great tool, it should be used wisely. Otherwise, mindless applications of great tools can result in the most pitiful outcomes. Let's not forget that our vision is analog, but our data is

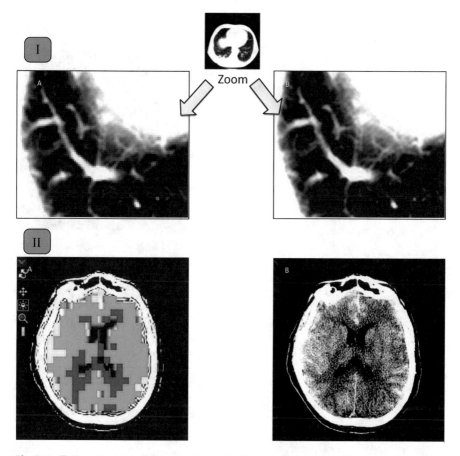

Fig. 3.6 (**I**) Zooming into a CT image: interactive (low-quality) *A*, changing into non-interactive but high-quality *B* when user finishes zooming adjustment (screenshots taken from AlgoM workstation, www.algom.com). (**II**) Zooming into MR image in a web client software: interactive (low-quality) image *A* is shown in a very detail-less, compressed way, to ensure real-time window/level adjustments; when the user finishes with the interactive work, image *B* is redrawn in full quality (AGFA web client)

digital. The only true way to achieve better display quality is to have better original images – acquired at higher resolution.

3.5   Math: Where Are Good Interpolation Techniques Coming From?

The word "math" would glaze the eyes of so many MI professionals that I sometimes wonder whether our perception of computers and informatics is well aligned with reality. So if you think that each computer contains a little green elf, solving problems with a wave of a little green wand, feel free to skip this chapter and

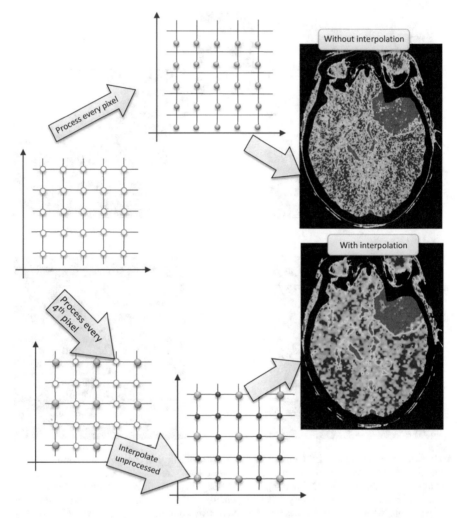

Fig. 3.7 Perfusion blood volume map, computed from the same perfusion image sequence without interpolation (*top*) and with interpolation (*bottom*). The use of interpolation results in a nearly 4x performance gain, but you can see the obvious drop in the image quality (resolution) in the interpolated case

the rest of the book. However, if you still believe that computers are nothing but math machines, using nothing but math to crunch our clinical projects, please keep reading. Math is not always easy, I know, but – believe me – dealing with the elves is much harder:)

So,

All interpolation methods are designed to excel at one single task: producing the highest interpolation quality for the broadest ranges of data. The rest, as always, depends on your definitions and priorities.

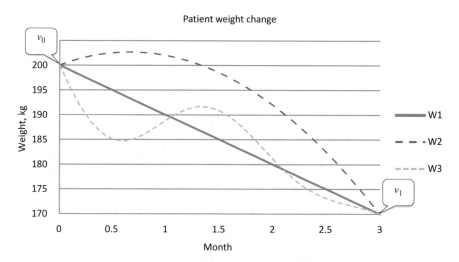

Fig. 3.8 Our imaginary weight loss program, with three possible weight loss functions W1, W2 and W3. Knowing the endpoints only, one cannot hypothesize about the most correct function choice, and therefore often resorts to the linear interpolation W1

Consider a patient whose weight at the beginning of your weight-loss experiment was 200 kg, which after three months dropped to 170. What was the patient's weight after the first month?

Let's count: the patient lost 10 kg/month on average, so we can assume that the patient's weight after the first month was $200 - 10 = 190$. Given that we did not make any other measurements, and have no idea of the monthly weight loss rate, 190 makes a reasonable approximation. This corresponds to the simplest and most frequently used linear interpolation, as we saw between pixels p_2 and p_3 in Fig. 3.1. In more strict terms, we can write linear interpolation between values v_0 and v_1 as

$$v(x) = v_0(1-x) + v_1 x$$
$$0 \leq x \leq 1$$
(3.1)

Here parameter x spans the distance between v_0 and v_1; $x=0$ corresponds to v_0 and $x=1$ corresponds to v_1. This means that $v(0)=v_0$, and $v(1)=v_1$ – as we mentioned, linear interpolation is exact at its endpoints. However, what happens in between, when $0<x<1$, is a much more intriguing question. What if the patient lost all 30 kg during the first week and kept the same weight after? Or what if the patient lost 40 kg, and then gained 10? Either scenario means some non-linear weight-change function, either makes sense, either is possible, but given v_0 and v_1 only, we just do not know anything else to make a more intricate, nonlinear formula (Fig. 3.8). So linear interpolation in Eq. (3.1) is the best we can do knowing only the two endpoints.

But if we do know something else about the weight-loss rate, we can generalize Eq. (3.1) as:

$$v(x) = v_0 h(x) + v_1 h(1-x)$$
$$0 \le x \le 1$$
(3.2)

where $h(x)$ is some function, known as the *interpolation kernel*; it defines how we mix the known endpoint values to find a value in between. Linear interpolation in Eq. (3.1) corresponds to the linear kernel $h_L(x) = 1-x$, but we know that other $h(x)$ are possible. The choice of $h(x)$ will depend on the additional information we might have about the weight-loss trends. Nonetheless, we still want $v(0) = v_0$ and $v(1) = v_1$, which takes us to the following

$$v(0) = v_0 h(0) + v_1 h(1-0) = v_0 h(0) + v_1 h(1) = v_0$$
$$v(1) = v_0 h(1) + v_1 h(1-1) = v_0 h(1) + v_1 h(0) = v_1$$
(3.3)

Since we assume that v_0 and v_1 can be anything, the only way to satisfy these two equations is to require

$$h(0) = 1, \quad h(1) = 0$$
(3.4)

You can see that these boundary conditions hold true for the linear kernel $h_L(x) = 1-x$. But they will be true for the some other $h(x)$ as well. Consider the nearest neighbor interpolation that we mentioned previously

$$h_{nn}(x) = \begin{cases} 1, & 0 \le x < 0.5 \\ 0, & 0.5 \le x < 1 \end{cases}$$
(3.5)

In our weight-loss experiment this means that the patient's weight stayed at 200 for the first half of the experiment (1.5 months), then dropped overnight to 170. This may sound a bit dramatic for a weight-loss program, but it definitely depends on the nature of your $v(x)$ function (consider plastic surgery or a magic laxative).

"Laxative? Wait a second!" – you should ask me by this time – "Isn't this supposed to be a digital imaging book? What do these weight-loss experiments have in common with digital image quality?? Are you plagiarizing from some late-night infomercial just to give your publishers enough to publish???"

Certainly not, my most attentive reader. And this is the whole point: interpolation techniques are universal, regardless of where they are applied. Pixels in digital images will be interpolated with exactly the same "weight-loss" equations we just covered, often using the simplest linear $h_L(x)$ in Eq. (3.1). But as we have already seen, simplest does not mean best, and we need more elaborate interpolation formulas to reflect more subtle weight... sorry, pixel intensity details. How can we develop these?

Surely by using more v_n points, and more complex $h(x)$. We can further generalize Eq. (3.2) as[6]

---

[6] Note that we added the requirement of symmetric kernels: $h(x) = h(-x)$.

$$v(x) = \sum_{n=1-N}^{N} v_n h(n-x)$$

(3.6)

$$0 \le |x| \le N, \quad h(x) = h(-x)$$

Here integer N stands for the *kernel support* size, which is the number of original points v_n that we want to use for interpolating the unknown $v(x)$. In the linear case we had $N=1$ (Eq. 3.1), but for the cubic pixel interpolation (enough of the weight loss allegories!) we will need $N=2$ (four points $\{p_1, p_2, p_3, p_4\}$ in Fig. 3.1). This generalization to any N uncovers two fundamental constraints on $h(x)$:

1. Consider all v_n equal to the same w, then $v(x)$ should be w as well, which leads to

$$w = \sum_{n=1-N}^{N} w h(n-x), \text{or}$$

(3.7)

$$\sum_{n=1-N}^{N} h(n-x) = 1 \quad \text{for any } 0 \le |x| \le N$$

This is known as the *partition of unity* requirement, and you can easily verify it for the linear $h_L(x)$ and nearest neighbor $h_{nn}(x)$ choices of $h(x)$.

2. Clearly, we want our interpolation in Eq. (3.6) to be exact at all endpoints v_n, meaning $v(n)=v_n$. This leads to generalized Eq. (3.4):

$$h(n) = \begin{cases} 1, & n = 0 \\ 0, & n \ne 0 \end{cases}$$

(3.8)

But this is really all we know about $h(x)$, and there are tons of kernels satisfying Eq. (3.7) – take $h_L(x)$ and $h_{nn}(x)$ as examples.

So here enters the most principal question in all of interpolation theory: given all possible choices of $h(x)$, can we propose the *best,* and what does "best" mean?

As previously mentioned, one of the most classical approaches to this problem is to build $h(x)$ which would be very accurate or even 100 % exact for broader classes of functions – in our case, for broader choices of pixel intensity-varying trends. Remember how we observed that $h_L(x)$ would be exact when pixel intensities follow the linear trend, but would fail for nonlinear (higher-order) trends? Can exact $h(x)$ go beyond linear? This problem of building a higher-order kernel was explored by Robert Keys in his 1981 paper (Keys 1981), presenting a very good example of interpolation design.

Keys searched for the best possible $h(x)$ assuming the following piecewise-cubic form[7]:

$$h_K(x) = \begin{cases} h_1(x) = A_1|x|^3 + B_1|x|^2 + C_1|x| + D_1, & 0 \le x < 1 \\ h_2(x) = A_2|x|^3 + B_2|x|^2 + C_2|x| + D_2, & 1 \le x < 2 \\ 0, & x \ge 2 \end{cases}$$

(3.9)

---

[7] Note how the formula uses the absolute value |x| to satisfy $h(x)=h(-x)$.

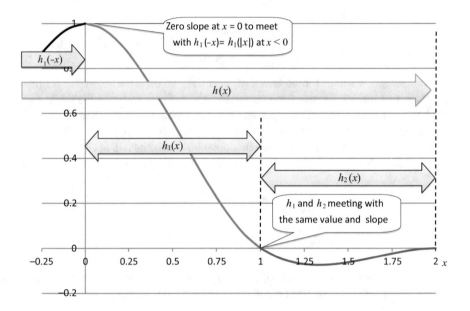

Fig. 3.9 Building Keys interpolation kernel $h_K(x)$ from two pieces $h_1(x)$ and $h_2(x)$. The coefficients of $h_1(x)$ and $h_2(x)$ were chosen to make cubic pieces meet at $x=0$ and $x=1$, at the same slope. Thus they formed a single smooth $h_K(x)$

In other words, Keys built his $h_K(x)$ from two cubic patches $h_1(x)$ and $h_2(x)$, stitched together at $x=0$ and $x=1$ (Fig. 3.9); this piecewise tactic gave him more freedom for building each piece. The stitching, along with conditions from Eqs. (3.7) and (3.8), led to a simple system of linear equations on the unknown coefficients in Eq. (3.9) (see the reference paper), which was solved leaving us with only one unknown parameter $a = A_2$:

$$h_K(x) = \begin{cases} h_1(x) = (a+2)|x|^3 - (a+3)|x|^2 + 1, & 0 \le x < 1 \\ h_2(x) = a|x|^3 - 5a|x|^2 + 8a|x| - 4a, & 1 \le x < 2 \\ 0, & x \ge 2 \end{cases} \qquad (3.10)$$

For any value of a, this produces a smooth continuous kernel $h_K(x)$, but this was not really our major point. As we mentioned earlier, interpolation is all about finding the optimal kernels, accurately interpolating broader classes of functions. Remember our linear interpolation $h_L(x)$ in Eq. (3.1)? If we use it to interpolate linear functions $v(x)$, the interpolation will be 100 % accurate (which is why we call linear a *first-order* interpolation). Keys wanted his $h(x)$ to be a *third-order* interpolation – that is, to be exact for any linear, quadratic, and cubic functions. Surprisingly

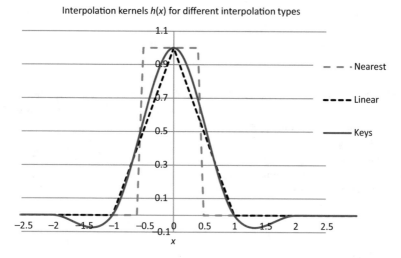

Fig. 3.10 Kernel function $h(x)$ for the nearest neighbor $h_{nn}(x)$, linear $h_L(x)$, and Keys $h_K(x)$ interpolations

enough, this can be done by setting $a = -1/2$ in Eq. (3.10), which was demonstrated by Keys in his work. Needless to say, this made Keys' kernel $h_K(x)$ far better than linear, and Eq. (3.10) – coined "bicubic interpolation" –a very popular choice in advanced digital image interpolation programs (Fig. 3.10).

Can we do better than Keys interpolation? We certainly can – the road to perfection is infinite. Using more polynomial "pieces" $h_i(x)$ in Eq. (3.9), and higher degrees of these polynomials will enable one to accurately interpolate more than cubic functions (Keys developed a fourth-order interpolation as well). Moreover, instead of high-order polynomial accuracy, one can use other different criteria of interpolation kernel optimality: highest order of approximation per given kernel "support size" N, minimal highest interpolation error (minmax problem), best preservation of the image frequency spectrum (image details), and so on. But as noted before, more elaborate interpolations become very pricey – they take longer to compute, and they need more points to process; Eq. (3.10) certainly looks more complex than Eq. (3.1). Therefore each particular problem – for example, interpolating certain classes of digital images – can easily lead to its own choice of the best interpolation kernel $h(x)$, designed to solve this particular task, and to achieve the best compromise between interpolation accuracy and computational performance.

I hope this little excursus into the land of optimal was not hard but helpful. If you are interested in more details on digital interpolation in medicine, I recommend reading Lehmann et al. (1999) and Unser (2000).

3.6   Self-check

3.6.1   Questions

1. In our example in Fig. 3.5, we used integer truncation, rounding decimal numbers *down* to the nearest integer. Although this is the default in computer math,[8]
   we can do better with rounding to the *nearest integer*: round(2.6)=3. Redo the
   Fig. 3.5 math using this approach. Observe the improvements, comparing your
   results to Fig. 3.5.
2. Estimate the fraction of interpolated pixels when displaying a full-screen MR
   image on your own computer/tablet/smartphone. Assume that MRI dimensions
   are smaller than those of your screen.
3. Verify (or, better, prove) Eq. (3.8), using Eq. (3.6).

3.6.2   Answers

1.

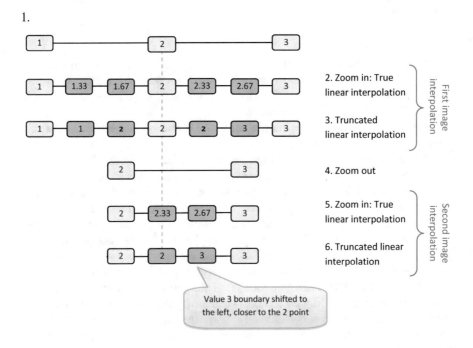

[8] For example, integer division like 14/3 would produce 4 in virtually all programing languages.
This is often referred to as "floor" truncation; for example, *floor*(2.6)=2.

2. Standard MRI image size is $N_{image} = 256 \times 256$ pixels, and if the resolution of your monitor is $W \times H$ pixels, full screen MRI will take $N_{screen} = min(W,H) \times min(W,H)$ of them (the largest square to fit the screen sizes). Therefore at least $(N_{screen} - N_{image})$ pixels will be interpolated, corresponding to the $F = 100 \times (1 - N_{image}/N_{screen})$ percent of the displayed image area. For example, consider a popular tablet with $W = 2,048$ and $H = 1,536$. Then $N_{screen} = 1,536 \times 1,536$ pixels, resulting in $F = 100 \times (1 - (256 \times 256)/(1,536 \times 1,536)) = 97\ \%$ percent of visible pixels coming from the interpolation algorithm, rather than from the original data.

References

Keys, R. G., 1981. Cubic Convolution Interpolation for Digital Image Processing. *IEEE Transactions on Acoustics, Speech, and Signal Processing,* pp. 1153–1160.

Lehmann, T. M., Gönner, C. & Spitzer, K., 1999. Survey: Interpolation Methods in Medical Image Processing. *IEEE Transactions on Medical Imaging,* pp. 1049–1075.

Pianykh, O. S., 2012. *DICOM: A Practical Introduction and Survival Guide.* Berlin, New York: Springer.

Pianykh, O. S., 2012. Finitely-supported L2-optimal kernels for digital signal interpolation. *IEEE Transactions on Signal Processing,* pp. 494–498.

Unser, M., 2000. Sampling-50 years after Shannon. *Proceedings of the IEEE,* pp. 569–587.

Image Compression

4

Key Points

Image compression is in constant demand as the only practical way to deal with ever-growing imaging data volume. *Lossless* compression does not change the original image, but achieves rather modest 2–4 compression factors. *Lossy* compression can typically reduce data volume by 10–20 times, but you need to be aware of the irreversible artifacts that it introduces into the images. This chapter explains the mechanics of compression and their impact on diagnostic imaging.

4.1 Why Even Bother?

Some 20 years ago, when I was starting my student research in image compression, my more advanced friends kept asking me, why on earth I chose to burden myself with such an antiquated and useless subject. Disk storage was growing rapidly, network bandwidth was rising, and dialup modems were firing data with "lightning-fast" 14 kb/s. Why compress, when we'll be able to handle everything uncompressed in a year?

But that year passed by, and then another, and by the time I joined my first Radiology department the folks around me were screaming from the data volume overdose. It turned out that the wonderful "larger storage, faster network" argument somehow missed its most essential counterpart: exploding data sizes. Clinical data volumes – medical imaging in particular, as the most megabyte-hungry – went through the hospital roofs, turning data storage and transmission into the most expensive enterprise of the digital age. Consequently, data compression has become an integral part of modern medical workflow, even if you never thought about it before. In fact, you can get yourself into serious trouble if you keep ignoring compression, as most of us did and still prefer to do. So let's spend some time studying how it works, and how it changes your diagnostic images.

O.S. Pianykh, *Digital Image Quality in Medicine*, Understanding Medical Informatics, 33
DOI 10.1007/978-3-319-01760-0_4, © Springer International Publishing Switzerland 2014

4.2   Lossless Compression

"Sure, I know how image compression works," you say. "It removes image pixels to make the image smaller!"

My dear interlocutor, you cannot even imagine how many times have I heard this brave answer. It's kind of natural to assume that to make something smaller you have to trim it down, but nothing could be further from reality in the case of image compression.

Contrary to popular belief, compression is the art of *rewriting the original information in the most condensed form*. Think about a hypothetical "Compressian" language, so laconic that translation into it always results in much shorter sentences and fewer letters. For example, imagine that you have a sequence S_1:

```
a a a a a b b b b b b b
```

which you "translate" into sequence S_2:

```
5a 7b
```

meaning that 'a' needs to be repeated five times, and 'b' – seven. Both sequences S_1 and S_2 are identical – they say exactly the same thing – but the second one is much shorter: you have 4 characters instead of the original 12, thus compressing the S_1 data with a 3:1 compression ratio.[1] This simple compression algorithm is known as *run-length encoding (RLE)* – we replace repetitive symbols (or numbers, or even entire words) by their counts. You may think that the example is a bit far-fetched; after all, who uses repetitive letters in a textual sentence? True enough, but who said that we have to compress text only? Think about images, where entire pixel lines may be equal to the same background color. Then instead of storing long sequences of identical pixels, we can apply RLE, instantly reducing the original data size.

As a result, RLE works great if the repetitive patterns are sequential. But one can do even better, exploring non-sequential redundancies. Moreover, you might be doing this daily without paying any attention to it. For instance, if you need to text sentence S_3:

```
You know that you are what you eat
```

and you don't have much time, you could type it as S_4:

```
u know that u r what u eat
```

which is definitely shorter than S_3. You simply picked the most frequently-used words – such as "you" and "are" – and replaced them with the shortest possible codewords, "u" and "r". Presto! You've built a simple compression dictionary (Table 4.1).

It's obvious that if you keep replacing the *most frequent* patterns with *shortest possible* codewords, you will shorten the data in the most efficient way; just make sure that your codewords are unique and cannot be parts of each other (a concept

---

[1] If we need to account for the spaces between the letters as well, then we get 23/5=4.6 compression.

Table 4.1 Simple compression dictionary	Original pattern	Codeword
	you	u
	are	r

known as *prefix coding*,[2] just as you see it in country calling codes). This is precisely what most frequency-based compression techniques do, whether it is LZW compression[3] used to make ZIP files, or Huffman compression[4] employed to compress images. These algorithms may rely on more advanced approaches to achieve the optimal encoding, but the essence of compression is the same: replacing the most redundant patterns with the shortest codewords does the job.

These trivial examples teach us a few valuable lessons:

– Compression attempts to encode the original data in the most compact form. This encoding is reversible: the original data can be fully recovered from its compressed representation (you can recover S_1 from S_2, or S_3 from S_4, without losing anything "in translation"). Therefore reversible compression is also known as *lossless*.
– Any compression is about exploring the original *data redundancy*. High redundancy (substantial presence of repetitive patterns) helps you achieve higher compression rates. Low redundancy (unpredictable patterns), on the contrary, makes data harder, if not impossible, to compress.
– Compression is quantified by compression ratio $R_C = \dfrac{\text{original data size}}{\text{compressed data size}}$. Thus, for our RLE example with S_1 and S_2, $R_c=3$.
– To translate the original into "Compressian", compression builds encoding dictionaries, replacing long repetitive patterns by short dictionary codewords. For instance, our dictionary in $\{S_3, S_4\}$ is shown in Table 4.1. Applying the dictionary in the reverse direction uncompresses S_4 back into S_3.
– Compression requires data processing: the computer has to find the most repetitive strings and replace them with the codewords; in some instances, it may have to compute the optimal codewords.[5] Processing takes time, and spending this time on compressing/uncompressing is the flip side of any compression implementation.

With these lessons learned, there is really nothing mind-blowing about the basic compression principles. Rest assured that none of them removes pixels from the original image data. Moreover, lossless compression can do a great job in many cases, with typical R_c ranging from 2 to 4. But this lossless idyll quickly fades when one runs into mega- and gigabytes of data (image databases, device raw data, high-resolution scans, large-scale projects). In this case we need at least an order of magnitude R_c before our workflow becomes remotely practical. We need to go *lossy*.

---

[2] http://en.wikipedia.org/wiki/Prefix_code

[3] See LZW on Wikipedia for a good example of its encoding.

[4] http://en.wikipedia.org/wiki/Huffman_coding

[5] You might have noticed that some compression software will offer you "normal" and "best" compression options, meaning that "best" will employ a more extensive search for redundant pieces.

4.3   Lossy Compression

One image pixel takes roughly the same memory as one letter. Now imagine that you have to store a CT image exam (500 images, for instance) along with some textual data of, say, 10,000 letters (patient demographics, history, report). Ten thousand letters may seem like a lot, but a standard 512×512 CT image has $512 \times 512 = 262,144$ pixels, which is already 26 times the size of the accompanying text. Now, if you multiply 26 by 500 images, you should get the full picture: medical images take a lot more space than medical text does.

So we need to target the images, and we need to compress them very efficiently. Just as we discussed earlier, images are sequences of pixels. One can read them line by line, starting from the top left pixel. Therefore lossy compression applies as usual: if we have a sequence S_5 of pixel values with something like:

1000 1000 1000 1003 1002 1005 1576 1623 1627 1620...

we can definitely apply RLE or LZW to compress it – for instance, replacing the values of 1000 with a shorter codeword "x" to build a compressed S_6:

3x 1003 1002 1005 1576 1623 1627 1620...

This looks good, but for most images this would yield R_c around 2: good enough to save on disk storage, but hardly enough to send that CT case to a smartphone in real-time, over a jammed network. Can we compress any stronger?

Yes, if we adopt the idea of irreversible *lossy compression*, achieving higher R_c through slight alterations in the original pixel values. Indeed, the difference between pixel values of 1000 and 1003 in S_5 may not have any diagnostic meaning. You may not even be able to perceive this difference at all. If this is the case, we can define a pixel error threshold ε – "perceptual error" – and consider all pixels within this threshold equal. For instance, if we choose $\varepsilon = 5$, then the original S_5 can be replaced by S_7 such that:

1000 1000 1000 1000 1000 1000 1576 1623 1623 1623...

This definitely increases the degree of redundancy, so that we can compress S_7 as S_8:

6x 1576 3y...

– a much better result compared to S_6.

> ▶ *Nota bene:* Note that in some cases, lossy compression is not an option. Consider text: we cannot pretend that the letters 'a' and 'b' are "close enough" to be interchangeable. We can afford to replace something only when the replacement doesn't matter to us.

Thus, lossy compression typically includes two distinct steps: approximating the original data samples with some admissible error ε to increase data redundancy, and compressing the approximate values with conventional lossless compression. When

Table 4.2 Summary of recommended compression rates in Canada, England, and Germany		Canada	England	Germany
	Radiography	20–30	10	10
	Mammography	15–25	20	15
	CT	8–15	5	5–8
	MR	16–24	5	7
	RF/XA	n/a	10	6

the approximation is exact ($\varepsilon=0$) we get our standard lossless case of nothing being lost or altered. It is when $\varepsilon>0$ that we lose the reversibility: one cannot recover S_5 from S_7.

Thus begins the whole "lossy vs. diagnostic" argument: how much ε round-off can we tolerate without losing diagnostic image quality? Think about setting $\varepsilon=700$ – then all ten pixel values in S_5 can be rounded to 1000, and the sequence will be compressed as 10x. This is a remarkably high compression ratio, but with all image detail totally lost! So we really want to stop somewhere in the middle between $\varepsilon=0$ and $\varepsilon=$"Gee, the image is gone!" – to preserve original diagnostic image quality while keeping the data size as small as possible.

This is exactly where lossy compression becomes more of an art. Suffice it to say that the differences between image pixel values can be diagnostic in some cases (such as tiny micro-calcifications in mammograms), and purely meaningless in others (such as noise in low-dose X-ray or CT images). Consequently, the same values of ε can be too high for one image (or image area, or specific malignancy) and way too low for another. Moreover, pixel value fluctuations can depend on different tissue types, image acquisition protocols, imaging artifacts, and so forth. As a result, there is no universally-perfect ε for diagnostically-safe lossy compression, and there is no universally-perfect R_c to ensure that your lossy image will stay flawless. Most literature on this matter seems to be strangely attracted to $R_c=10$, but some suggest 15–20 (Kim et al. 2012), 70 (Peterson and Wolffsohn 2005), or even $R_c=171$ (Peterson et al. 2012),[6] while the others advise caution even at $R_c=8$ (Erickson et al. 2010) – always specific to the images, circumstances, experiences[7] or even countries (Table 4.2) (Loose et al. 2009), without any guarantee that the same R_c will work for you. This leaves you with only one real option: trying it yourself. If you are using lossy compression – inevitable in projects like teleradiology – you *will* need to experiment with different compression settings provided in your software to see that the diagnostic integrity of your images remains intact.[8]

---

[6] Apart from compression, the authors also used several image format conversion steps (DICOM, BMP, AVI) which could have made image quality even worse.

[7] I can tell from my own experience that older radiologists seem to be more tolerant to image artifacts, and some publications confirm this point (Erickson et al. 2010).

[8] Don't ask your software vendor – why would they care?

▶ *Nota bene:* Keep in mind that there is absolutely no straightforward way to associate compression ratio R_c with compressed image quality; the latter depends on many objective and subjective factors such as image texturing or human vision phenomena, generally ignored by the compression algorithms. But compression ratio works perfectly well when we talk about data size reduction – this is precisely what R_c means, and this is why it is so much appreciated.

To carry out this task of identifying compression artifacts, we need to look at them more closely.

4.4   JPEG Artifacts

JPEG compression and image format have been around since the 1990s, and have gained enormous popularity with many applications, including early adoption by the DICOM standard (Pianykh 2005). Instead of ε-thresholding that we discussed earlier, JPEG takes a different route. First, it breaks an image into 8×8 blocks to localize image features, and approximates each block in 2D by representing it as a weighted sum of predefined 8×8 intensity patterns ("codewords", based on Discrete Cosine Transform functions, or DCT,[9] Fig. 4.1). Then, instead of storing the original $8 \times 8 = 64$ pixel values in each block, JPEG needs to store only a few weighting coefficients, required for the block's DCT decomposition – and that's how the compression magic is done. This is a good way to explore image redundancies: first of all, we take full advantage of the 2D image format; second, naturally-smooth images will require only a few top DCT coefficients per block, leading to high compression ratios.

Inversely, when the images get noisy, or block boundaries run across some image edges (such as sharp intensity changes between different organs), JPEG magic starts falling apart. And when this happens, JPEG's 8×8 blocks will be right in your face – then you'll know the tiger by its tail. Why does JPEG have this artifact? To achieve high R_c, JPEG has to sacrifice the heaviest ballast of its higher-order DCT coefficients, the ones responsible for the fine image details. Thus, only the less numerous, least-detailed patterns survive, resulting in dull and disconnected checkerboards (Fig. 4.2, right).

It's important to know that the JPEG compression standard has several advanced flavors, lossless included. You can find them in DICOM software (often used on CT and MR scanners), but they won't be supported in popular imaging applications such as web browsers or image editors. So bear in mind that using JPEG in your online photo album will always imply baseline lossy compression – even if you set JPEG image quality to the highest possible.

---

[9] In essence, DCT is the "cosine" part of the Fourier transform – thanks to Jean Baptiste Fourier, brave Napolean officer and governor of Low Egypt. See more at http://en.wikipedia.org/wiki/Discrete_cosine_transform

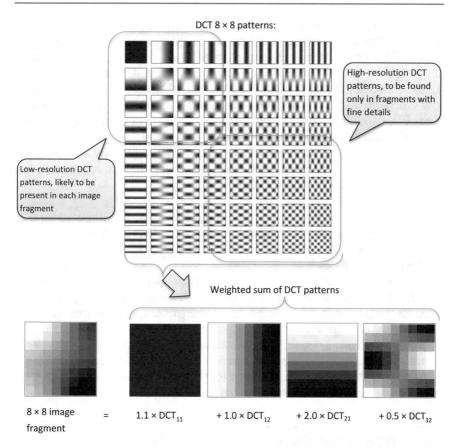

Fig. 4.1 JPEG uses predefined DCT image patterns to represent each 8×8 fragment of the original image. If we can approximate the fragment with only a few DCT patterns, then all we need to store is the pattern coefficients, such as $\{1.1, 1.0, 2.0, 0.5\}$ in our example. Storing those few coefficients instead of the original 64 pixels is the key idea behind JPEG compression

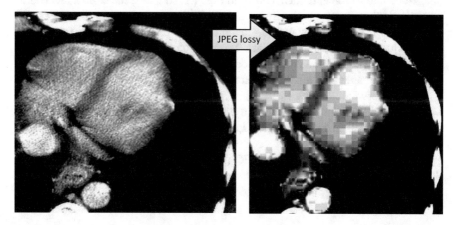

Fig. 4.2 Too much of JPEG's lossy compression will leave you with severe blocking artifacts. Note that all fine texture details, present in the original image (*left*), are gone in the compressed image (*right*). $R_c = 20$

In addition to that and probably due to its venerable age, JPEG supports only 8-bit and 12-bit pixel grayscales. This means that you can have only up to $2^8 = 256$ or $2^{12} = 4{,}096$ shades of gray in your medical image, depending on the flavor of JPEG you are using. DICOM, on the contrary, supports deeper 16-bit grayscale. This matters because putting a DICOM image into JPEG may bring to mind that old joke Procrustes played on his unfortunate guests. If you want to store a 16-bit-deep X-ray in a standard browser-compatible 8-bit JPEG, you will have chop off half of the original image grayscale depth, $8 = 16 - 8$ bits. In plain terms it means that each 256 shades of the original image will be collapsed into a single procrustean shade of your JPEG. This will certainly wipe out many diagnostic features; don't be surprised if you get a single color per body part.

▶ *Nota bene:* Keep in mind that compression is yet another application layer added to your imaging workflow. As such, it may have problems of its own – and oh, yes! – its own bugs. I have seen hospitals where poor JPEG implementations were simply corrupting the images.

Why this is possible, you may ask? Writing compression code is not easy, and requires substantial subject expertise. Therefore most vendors prefer to get prêt-à-porter compression libraries. You can either buy them from professional companies (which implies costs and royalties), or adopt some (nearly-) free public solutions. The latter are typically found online, or borrowed from research projects that were never meant to work on a commercial-grade scale. So after processing 1000 images successfully, they inevitably fail on image 1001, simply because their original developers (long gone) never thought of testing this many.

4.5   JPEG2000 Artifacts

JPEG2000 compression, just as its name suggests, appeared on the wake of the new millennium, as a "new generation" JPEG. Just like JPEG, JPEG2000 takes the same image-decomposition approach, shown in Fig. 4.1, so that it can store a few coefficients instead of many pixels. But unlike its DCT-driven predecessor, JPEG2000 decomposes images with wavelets – another set of cleverly designed functions – invented to represent feature-rich data. The key point about wavelets is their ability to capture local image details (such as edges and little structures) without artificially breaking the images into the 8×8 blocks.

This property, along with many other mathematically-optimal properties of the wavelet transform, made JPEG2000 a long-awaited compression favorite; and it does do very well in many medical apps. Moreover, JPEG2000 has no problem accommodating 16-bit pixels of your medical DICOM images, with lossy image quality usually superior to that of JPEG (Shiao et al. 2007; Gulkesen et al. 2010). But as always, overdoing its lossy compression leads to diagnostically-unacceptable artifacts, shown in Fig. 4.3; instead of JPEG's blocking, JPEG2000 can result in

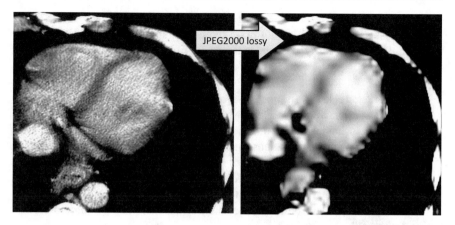

Fig. 4.3 Overdoing lossy JPEG2000 results in blur with blobbing around the edges. $R_c = 20$

substantial image blur. It happens for the same reasons: when JPEG2000 has to achieve high R_c, it starts sacrificing the fine local details, as taking the most memory to store. The strategy inevitably results in blurred, detail-less areas, very much like we saw with our good old friend, JPEG.

Another theoretically useful functionality explored by JPEG2000 authors was the ability to encode and stream different image regions using different strengths of compression (R_c). It was expected that this would significantly reduce the volume of data being downloaded: if the user is only going to look at a specific area, only this area needs to be transmitted with the highest quality. Unfortunately, this approach proved to be somewhat controversial: as more and more regions and details were streamed to the user, the image on the user side would keep updating itself, changing in quality and resolution. Virtually any radiologist would prefer to have the final image first, before even glancing at it.

4.6   JPEG-LS and Diagnostic Compression

Remember our initial discussion about the pixel error threshold ε used in lossy compression? Well, as you can tell by now, it is not the only lossy approach and, to be exact, it is not even the one used by JPEG and JPEG2000. And as a result of this, JPEG and JPEG2000 can control lossy image quality only through the choice of the overall compression ratio R_c: *on average*, but not at each pixel. This is not really good news for your diagnostic imaging: you simply do not know where this average error can sweep to its highest extremes and what important image features this may erase.

This shortcoming was taken into account by the authors of the JPEG-LS compression algorithm, which does rely on ε thresholding to control compression loss at each pixel (Weinberger et al. 2005). Thus, for $\varepsilon = 0$ we have a completely lossless compression – all pixel intensities stay unchanged. For $\varepsilon > 0$ the algorithm becomes lossy – or, because of its tight grip on each pixel's value, *nearly-lossless*.

▶ *Nota bene:* Being able to go from lossless to lossy with the same algorithm is another practical advantage of JPEG-LS. Believe it or not, this is not possible with all image compression techniques. JPEG, for instance, uses very different algorithms for its lossless and lossy implementations, and there are *18 types* (!) of JPEG algorithms, new and retired, included in DICOM for medical image compression. This variety only adds to confusion ("Which JPEG am I using?") and complexity (implementing several versions of JPEG to support different compression types). As we all understand, any confusion or complexity inevitably invites more bugs, corrupted data, and incompatible applications.

JPEG-LS was standardized and adopted by DICOM just like its other JPEG siblings, yet it is very much unknown anywhere else. Its original page at www.hpl.hp.com/research/info_theory/loco/ still remains the main source for curious minds. Nonetheless, JPEG-LS fit well in the realm of diagnostic imaging, for two principal reasons: controlling lossy error at each pixel, and working fast. The ε error threshold gives us a truly diagnostic compression: one usually knows how many intensity levels can be tweaked safely, without altering the diagnostic value of the image. Besides, even keeping ε very low ($\varepsilon = 1$ or $\varepsilon = 2$) can provide you with higher-than-lossless R_c, while making only perceptually-invisible alterations (hence another name, *perceptually-lossless* compression). In short, having JPEG-LS in your compression arsenal is a safe and practical option.

But is JPEG-LS artifact-free? Certainly yes for $\varepsilon = 0$, and certainly no for $\varepsilon > 0$. Even the best possible lossy compression, when abused, can result in very visible distortions. Figure 4.4 illustrates the JPEG-LS artifact pattern, although I had to ramp ε up to 21 to make it visible at all. Overdosing on JPEG-LS clearly produces horizontal streaks, which look entirely unnatural and annoying (definitely worse than JPEG2000 blur). Can you guess where they're coming from?

You can, if you still remember the use of RLE compression in the lossy case, as we discussed a bit earlier. JPEG-LS processes image pixels line by line, and when several pixels on a line have the same intensity within the ε threshold, JPEG-LS switches to the RLE mode, setting the pixels to the same exact value. This is precisely how we compressed S_5 to S_8 a few pages back, using S_7 as a nearly-lossless equivalent of S_5. But this led to six equal pixels at the beginning of S_7, which is exactly the "same-color" streak artifact seen in Fig. 4.4.

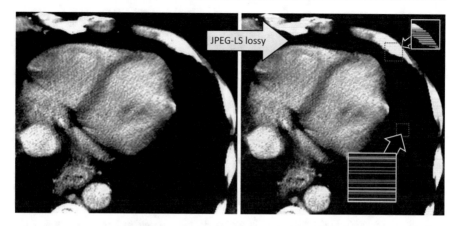

Fig. 4.4 Overdoing lossy JPEG-LS leads to visible streaking artifacts (horizontal lines with constant pixel intensity). The streaking comes from the RLE, when several pixels along the same line get rounded to the same value. This is particularly true for the areas where pixel values are originally close, such as a dark image background; the *inserts* show these patterns with higher contrast. Nonetheless, the soft tissue area in the center was preserved much better with JPEG-LS than with compatible JPEG and JPEG2000 compression. Same $R_c = 20$, $\varepsilon = 21$

In other words, we got the streaks not because of some JPEG-LS failure, but because we assumed that $\varepsilon = 21$ would be a diagnostically-safe error, and it is clearly not.

So here comes the résumé: the artifacts shown in Figs. 4.2, 4.3 and 4.4 were very visible because we made them such, targeting relatively high $R_c = 20$. This should not discourage you from using lossy compression wisely: you wouldn't see any of these problems at $R_c = 10$. But knowing the visual artifact patterns should provide you with very valuable hints on how your images might be, or might have been compressed.

▶ *Nota bene:* As we know by now, any damage to a digital image is permanent: once done, it cannot be reversed. So if images have been over-compressed elsewhere, even before reaching your PACS or diagnostic workstation, they are already infested with the artifacts regardless of what happens to them next. And the more rounds of lossy compression they undergo, the worse it gets – just like faxing a faxed copy of a faxed document will make it completely illegible. Therefore if you do employ lossy compression, make sure you know when and how often it takes place for each image. I have seen software that uses lossy every time when saving images to a disk. Now you know what that can amount to.

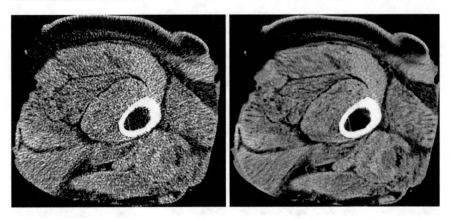

Fig. 4.5 Natural noise in CT data – high in the low-dose image (*left*) and lower in high-dose CT (*right*)

4.7   Compression and Image Quality

The relationship between lossy image compression and diagnostic image quality is not as trivially inverse as it might appear at first. Let me give you a few examples.

Consider noise – a random variability in image pixel values that comes naturally in all image acquisition devices. Because of its random nature, noise is impossible to compress; it has no patterns, no redundancies to take advantage of. For that reason, noise has always been the principal enemy of data compression: you cannot achieve high R_c with noisy data.

On the other hand, noise is the principal enemy of diagnostic image interpretation as well: it occludes important details; it simply pollutes the image (Fig. 4.5). This points us to a couple of interesting ideas:

- What we lose by applying lossy compression may not be so important. Sometimes it may be just pure, useless noise. When lossy compression threshold $\varepsilon > 0$ happens to be close to that of the natural pixel noise, the compression alterations will stay hidden in the noise, without touching anything diagnostic. Fritsch and Brennecke (2011) make this argument to demonstrate that lossy JPEG with $R_c = 10$ can be used safely with digital X-ray images; not because they still "look kinda good" (precarious and subjective statement), but because JPEG loss at $R_c = 10$ stays close to the level of loss associated with the natural X-ray noise (Fig. 4.6).
- Removing noise from the images can benefit both their diagnostic value and compressibility (Gupta et al. 2005). For example, the past decade was all about low-dose CT imaging. Scores of clever filters were developed to remove CT noise from the low-dose scans, making them look like high-dose CTs. But indirectly, the same filters improved image compressibility. Sure, you can't really call lossy compression a noise-removal tool; you need a set of totally different algorithms to do it right. But it is not unfeasible to design a noise-removal algorithm that will improve diagnostic image quality and reduce compressed image size at the same time.

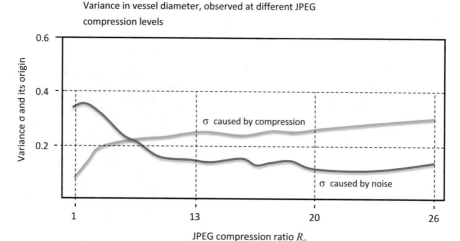

Fig. 4.6 Variance σ observed in 3 mm vessel diameter on phantom coronary angiography images, based on Fritsch and Brennecke (2011) results. For relatively low compression ratio R_c, the original X-ray noise dominates the lossy compression artifacts. As R_c increases, lossy compression begins to smooth out the original noise, and introduce more pronounced artifacts of its own

And noise is only one example of a diagnostically worthless image component that can be suppressed to improve compression ratios. There are many others – take pitch-black image background (Fig. 4.5), which still contains a lot of pixels that we need to store and transmit without ever putting them to any good use. Had all background pixels had the same intensity value (0, for instance), JPEG-LS or JPEG2000 would have removed them in the most optimal way. Unfortunately this is not the case; natural noise and natural acquisition aberrations make background pixels slightly different from each other. If we knew that we could safely set all these pixels to 0, we could make significant improvements in R_c, such as the 40–58 % increase that has been reported for CT background removal in (Kim et al. 2011). Furthermore, consider different tissues and organs, which may have different diagnostic importance, especially in the context of a particular study. This importance can be related to the error threshold ε, used by lossy compression algorithms. Instead of using the same ε for the entire image, one can assign higher ε to the least important pixels, and lower ε to the most important. In this case, diagnostic value becomes the major criterion for "losing" in lossy compression, and lossy compression can indeed work as an image-enhancing technique, deliberately "losing" diagnostically-irrelevant jumble –provided, of course, that you can develop an efficient metric to compute this diagnostic ε automatically (Fig. 4.7).

These non-trivial effects should only reinforce our previous statement: the only way to evaluate any lossy compression is to check it with your bare eyes, in the context of your quality expectations. If your lossy-compressed images look 100 % perfect, you might even consider compressing them further. However, if you start seeing compression artifacts, you need to reduce your compression appetite. No one will make this decision for you.

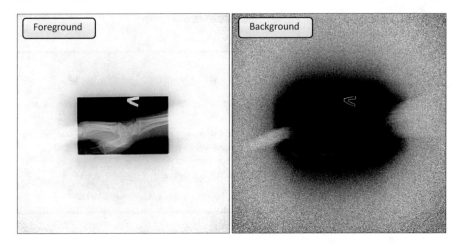

Fig. 4.7 Noise in medical images. *Left*: The original image. *Right*: The same image with a different intensity window, set to show the background pixels. You can see that the background, which appears uniformly gray in the left image, actually consists of purely noisy pixel values

▶ *Nota bene:* By the way, how do you know whether your images are compressed? There are several ways to figure this out:

- Visible artifacts, as discussed
- Various signs in your program interface. In most countries it is required to indicate that medical images have undergone lossy compression.

Image file sizes. For instance, a standard 512×512 CT has 2 bytes per image pixel, so its DICOM file size should be around $512 \times 512 \times 2$ bytes, or 500 KB. It might be a bit larger because of the text tags included in the file, but if you see a 250 KB or 70 KB size instead, you definitely have a compressed CT. Moreover, you can guess whether the compression was lossy using $R_c = 3$ as a reasonable lossless threshold. Thus, in our CT example, a 250 KB file corresponds to $R_c = 500/250 = 2$, which is indicative of lossless compression. A 70 KB CT file size means $R_c = 500/70 = 7$, which strongly suggests lossy compression; start watching for the artifacts.

4.8   Compression Pitfalls

The two principal reasons for using image compression are to save disk space and to increase image transmission speed.

The disk space reduction is pretty straightforward: if you can compress the images with $R_c = 3$, you will store three images instead of one. This immediately translates into money saved on expanding your digital archive. These days, many hospitals are trying to store all the images they acquire, under the ambitious "keep everything forever" imperative. This starts getting costly, and it is generally assumed that at least the most aged images can be stored with lossy compression, since their significance for the current patient interpretation decreases with time.

The only problems with compression used for long-term storage are the inevitable changes in compression algorithms, and the slew of proprietary compression implementations from different vendors. Most vendors – keep this in mind – do not write their own image compression code. They prefer to purchase it from smaller companies, absorbing the entire businesses and replacing the original development teams. This results in countless discontinuities in the original product content and implementation, and equally countless algorithmic changes in data storage routines. As a result, when you have to migrate to another vendor (such as a different PACS[10] archive solution), you may discover that the images you so conveniently compressed some 10 years ago cannot be uncompressed by your new PACS provider, just because "it's been a while" and "we don't support this anymore". So when considering a new vendor, always check your compression for compatibility. It's easy to do – just try to open your compressed images with another vendor's software (one that claims to use the same type of image compression algorithm), and see what happens.

Compression for faster image networking is another popular myth that needs to be taken with a good grain of salt. As we mentioned earlier, compression is computationally intensive: the computer has to scan long data sequences, locate the most repetitive patterns, and replace them with shorter codewords. This takes processing time. So consider this example: if it takes you 10 seconds to transmit and someone offers you the option to compress your images with some impressive $R_c = 10$, would you gain anything from this compression? The typical answer is, "Sure, we'll reduce our transmission time from 10 to 1 second $(1 = 10/R_c)$", but this is a *wrong* answer. You may enable a compression option only to discover that it takes 5 seconds to compress the volume on the sender side, and another 5 seconds to uncompress it on the receiver side, which is already the 10 seconds that the entire uncompressed transmission was taking! As a result, compression can easily make your networking *slower*, and, if lossy, your images *worse*; a lose-lose outcome of less-than-thoughtful compression implementation. The only way to avoid this is to time your networking with compression set on and off, to determine the best option empirically.

Finally, keep in mind that the main idea behind the lossy compression was our inability to perceive some small pixel changes. But as digital image volumes continue to skyrocket, more and more diagnostic tasks will be delegated to CAD (Computer-Aided Diagnostics). Unlike human eyes, computers *will* perceive the smallest pixel deviations, and 1000 *will not* look like 1001 to them. This means two things:

– Lossy compression can affect the quality of CAD. Researchers from the University of Mainz in Germany (Ridley 2011) reported a 20 % increase in false CAD results at $R_c = 15$, and (Raffy et al. 2006) reported their CAD breakdown[11] around $R_c = 48$.
– In computer applications, the permissible lossy compression error ε should be chosen based on the algorithm's sensitivity to errors, and not on human perception. This is only the only way to ensure the objectivity of ε selection.

---

[10] Picture Archiving and Communication System, major application for working with diagnostic images.

[11] The CAD was used to detect lung nodules.

▶ *Nota bene:* Note that all lossy image compression algorithms work only with local pixel intensity approximations, and do not take into any account other intensity-related features such as image textures. CAD, in contrast, gets very particular about texturing patterns. Lossy compression does change image texturing. In fact, the artifacts we observed with lossy JPEG, JPEG2000, and JPEG-LS can be viewed as texturing artifacts, and therefore will affect CAD outcomes.

Alas, but this is the nature of any advanced technology: the more complex it becomes, the more weight you will feel on your shoulders. But the gains can be impressive as well, so be brave and explore your options.

4.9   Compression vs. Interpolation

Just for the fun of it, let us revisit that old myth of the "pixel removing" compression, mentioned at the beginning of our brief compression journey. What would happen to image quality had we actually considered removing image pixels to reduce image size?

Let's grab our favorite example, a CT image with 512×512 pixels. The only reasonable way to "remove pixels" from it would be to reduce its resolution. Thus, downsampling the image by a factor of $f=2$, we would scale the CT down to 256×256 pixels – a quarter of the original image size – and permanently lose three-quarters of the original pixel data. This would be equivalent to lossy compression with $R_c=4$, provided we can somehow "uncompress" the downsampled image. How do we turn a 256×256 image back into a 512×512 one?

There is only one way to do this, and you know it already: interpolation. In other words, interpolation can be used as a very simple-minded lossy "decompression", compensating for the lossy "compression" based on pixel removal.

Would it work better compared to true compression? I think you should be able to guess the answer by now, but Fig. 4.8 gives you a more solid illustration. We used JPEG2000 lossy compression, comparing the loss in JPEG2000 to that caused by image downsampling followed by cubic interpolation. The loss in the images was measured as mean square error from the original image. As you can see, $R_c=25$ produced visible blur in JPEG2000, but it looks like nothing compared to the total destruction caused by interpolated downsampling. This result was completely anticipated, and yet it is worth looking at. First of all, it teaches us yet another lesson about the dangers of digital image resizing – that interpolation cannot compensate for the loss of the original image data, nor can it be used as a substitute for image compression. Second, it shows that the effort and time invested in advanced image compression techniques were not wasted; and although we should remain cautious about the use of lossy in diagnostic imaging, we can certainly use it wisely to keep our data clinically sound.

Errors from compression and interpolation

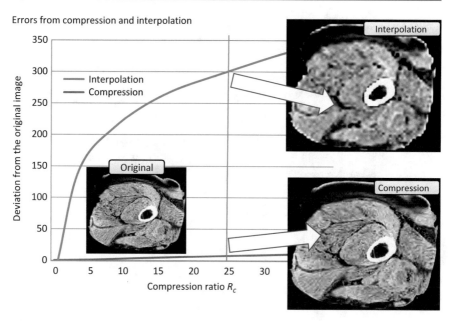

Fig. 4.8 Comparing changes in the original data produced by interpolation and lossy image compression. *Interpolation*: the original image was downsampled at different factors *f*, and then restored back to the original resolution with cubic interpolation. *Compression*: the original image was compressed with lossy JPEG2000. For each approach, mean square error was computed to measure image deviation from the original. The image *inserts* show the results for the interpolated (*top*) and compressed (*bottom*) images at $R_c = 25$; the image on the *left* is the original

4.10   Informatics: Where Good Image Compression Is Coming From?

Although the principal concepts of image compression are very straightforward and easy to grasp, may I invite you to take a bit deeper dive into their most colorful reefs? This should help you appreciate the ingenuity of compression algorithm developers.

One can certainly compress images with generic compression algorithms such as ZIP, but this will miss the most important thing: the image-specific data format. Very much *unlike* sentences, digital images are two-dimensional,[12] and each image pixel is surrounded by its pixel neighbors. With a few exceptions for high noise and inter-object boundaries, all neighboring pixels tend to have very similar intensities. This similarity makes pixel data more predictable, and one can use a few nearest neighbors to estimate the next adjacent pixel value. That is, predictable means redundant, and hence more compressible. And this is precisely what all advanced image compression algorithms exploit to the finest extremes.[13]

---

[12] Can be 3D and higher for volumetric and more complex imaging data.

[13] Contrast this with RLE compression, which simply assumes that the next pixel in line has the same value as its predecessor.

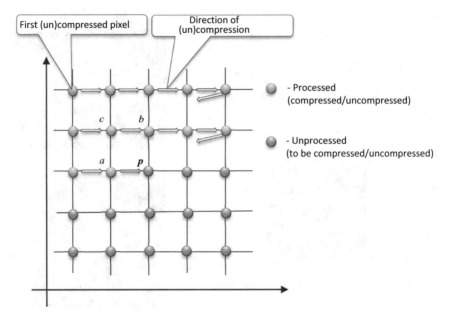

Fig. 4.9 Image compression, taking advantage of 2D image format. Both compressing and uncompressing passes will process pixel data line by line, using already known neighbor values *a*, *b*, *c* to process the next pixel value *p*

As a result, the first step in virtually any image compression technique, lossless in particular, would be the use of *predictive models*, taking advantage of the neighboring pixel similarity. An image is compressed and uncompressed pixel-by-pixel and line-by-line, starting from the top-left corner (Fig. 4.9). This means that by the time we need to compress or uncompress current pixel *p*, we would already have processed its neighbors *a*, *b* and *c*. Can we use these three neighbors to improve *p*'s compression?

We can. Assuming pixel value similarity, one can observe that $p + c$ should be somewhat close to $a + b$, thus making $a + b - c$ a good estimate for *p*:

$$\hat{p} = a + b - c \quad \text{(predicted value of } p\text{)}$$
$$p = \hat{p} + \delta = a + b - c + \delta \quad \text{(true value of } p\text{)} \quad\quad (4.1)$$
$$\delta = p - \hat{p} = p - a - b + c \quad \text{(prediction error)}$$

Here $\hat{p}$ is the predicted value of *p*, built from the known neighbors *a*, *b* and *c*. This prediction cannot be perfectly exact, and residual $\delta = p - \hat{p}$ will reflect the prediction error, the only part we really do not know about *p*. And, more interestingly, δ can be used *instead* of *p*, both in compressing and uncompressing processes:
- When we reach pixel *p* while *compressing* the image, we know *p*'s value and can find δ as $p - a - b + c$ (Eq. 4.1). Then instead of compressing and storing the original *p*, we can compress and store its residual δ.

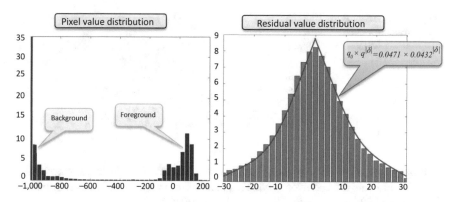

Fig. 4.10 Comparing the frequencies of the original pixel values and their residuals. Horizontal axis shows the values, and vertical – frequency percentages. *Left*: Typical distribution of original pixel intensities p in a CT image. *Right*: Distribution of predictive residuals δ in the same image

- Conversely, when we reach pixel p while *uncompressing* the image, we do not know p yet, but we can use stored and uncompressed δ to recover it as $p = a + b - c + \delta$.

Why would this strange pixel trickery matter? Well, think about it – we expect close pixels to have close values. That is, we expect δ values to be much smaller in magnitude than the original p. Then:

- Smaller residuals δ will take fewer bits to store, so keeping them instead of p already opens a path to a more efficient compression.
- The distribution of δ values will follow a better-defined pattern. In particular, due to pixel similarity, we expect smaller δ values to be more frequent. Knowing δ distribution eliminates the need to search for the most frequent patterns, a process so time-consuming in all data compression algorithms. We gain performance.

I illustrate this with Fig. 4.10, built from a typical CT image. The left side of the figure shows a classic distribution of the original pixel intensities, which would usually fall into background and foreground intensity clusters. As you can see, the range of p values is extremely wide, and the distribution pattern – too complex to suggest any *ad hoc* encoding vocabulary. On the contrary, the right side of the figure shows a very compact and well-shaped distribution of the corresponding δ residuals, peaking around $\delta = 0$ as we expected. Moreover, it was empirically observed that the δ distribution can be very closely approximated with two-sided geometric distribution (TSGD) of the form $q_0 \times q^{|\delta|}$, where q_0 and q are some constants. And finally, it was discovered that the optimal codeword dictionary for TSGD follows a very simple Golomb code pattern: 1, 01, 001, 0001, ... (Golomb 1966).[14] That is, the most frequent residual value $\delta = 0$ should be encoded with a single bit 1, the next frequent $\delta = -1$ with two bits 01, the next $\delta = 1$ – with 001 and so on, as shown in Table 4.3:

---

[14] See http://en.wikipedia.org/wiki/Golomb_coding

Residual value δ	Codeword, bits
0	1
−1	01
1	001
−2	0001
2	00001
−3	000001
...	...

Table 4.3 Codewords to encode residual values, used in JPEG-LS

Binary Golomb code is nothing but "comma-separated" codewords, where bit 1 is used to indicate the codeword end. This makes Golomb code easy to program and fast to process. If your residual sequence looked like S_δ:

0 0 1 0 −3 .....

then its Golomb-compressed version will be S_G:

110011000001

You may have a couple of questions at this point:

- Why is compressed S_G longer than the original S_δ? It is not. Recall that the original residuals were in integer format, meaning that each number in S_δ is stored with standard integer precision – typically 16 bits per pixel in DICOM image format. So five residuals in S_δ take $5 \times 16 = 80$ bits. S_G, on the contrary, is a bit sequence, taking exactly the 12 bits it contains. Thus, in our example S_G will use $80/12 = 6.7$ times less storage than S_δ.
- If we merged all codewords into a single S_G sequence, would we always be able to split it back into the same codewords? Yes, Golomb coding is an example of *prefix coding* mentioned earlier, where no codeword can be a beginning of another codeword. In the case of Golomb coding it's rather obvious: we use bit 1 as a separator between the codewords. Had we used codeword 0 for $\delta = 1$ in Table 4.3, we would have been in trouble: 001 could mean "0 and 01" or "0, 0 and 1", and we wouldn't be able to decode S_G uniquely. See how tiny details can make big differences?

In short, the wonderful and nontrivial mix of 2D image format, predictive models and coding ingenuity leads to a far more efficient compression scheme, and superior compression ratios.

Can it be improved any further?

Yes, but you'll have to weigh the cost of such improvement against image quality and performance. First, nearly-lossless compression with ε thresholding can easily be added to this model, if we round all δ residuals with $\pm \varepsilon$ precision:

$$\delta' = sign(\delta) \left\lfloor \frac{|\delta| + \varepsilon}{2\varepsilon + 1} \right\rfloor \tag{4.2}$$

where $\lfloor . \rfloor$ means rounding down to the nearest integer. For threshold $\varepsilon = 0$, this equation will not change anything: $\delta' = sign(\delta)|\delta| = \delta$. But $\varepsilon > 0$ will shrink the range of δ' values proportionally, reducing large δ, and increasing the number of δ' close to 0. This will result in predominantly shorter Golomb sequences, and even better compression – at the cost of "nearly-lossless" loss (Fig. 4.11).

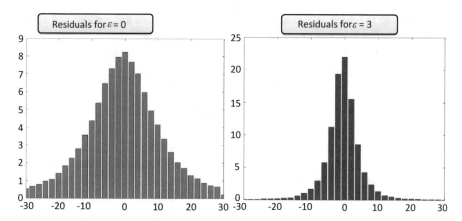

Fig. 4.11 Change in δ residual distribution pattern (residual values are given along the horizontal axis, and their frequency in % – along the vertical one). *Left*: Distribution of residuals for $\varepsilon=0$, lossless compression. *Right*: Distribution of residuals for $\varepsilon=3$, lossy compression. Note that lossy residuals have much tighter distribution around $\delta=0$, which leads to predominantly shorter Golomb codewords and better compression

Second, one can come up with more intricate predictors in lieu of (Eq. 4.1) – using more than three pixel neighbors, for instance. In theory, more complex predictors should provide higher prediction accuracy, leading to even smaller and more compressible δ values. However, the improvements in compression ratio R_c may be negligible, while the performance cost for computing more complex formulas is high. This is the point where many compression algorithm developers will have to compromise, usually leaning toward simpler but more efficient techniques. Beware of any time-consuming compression – in some cases it can only make your imaging worse (see self-check problems below).

I hope that our little compression discussion has made you more compression-aware. I also hope that it might save you from reinventing the wheel – experimenting with blackening image background or smoothing images to prove that this improves their compressibility. It certainly does so, as it increases data redundancy, but this is a trivial point. Objective, fast, and diagnostically safe image compression is still a far more interesting challenge to tackle.

4.11 Self-check

4.11.1 Questions

1. You need to start a teleradiology project, sending CT images to a remote clinic for reports. You have measured the network link speed to that clinic; it is 10 MB/s on average. So you consider image compression as a way to send the images faster. The compression software you have takes 2 seconds to compress (or uncompress) 100 CT images, with average $R_c=3.2$. Is it worth using compression, and why?

CT image size is 0.5 MB. Show any calculations supporting your decision.

2. Assuming the same setup, what needs to be done to make the compressed image exchange twice as fast as uncompressed?
3. JPEG-LS improves (Eq. 4.1) with the following pixel predictor for $\hat{p}$:

$$\hat{p} = \begin{cases} \min(a,b), & \text{if } c \geq \max(a,b) \\ \max(a,b), & \text{if } c \leq \min(a,b) \\ a+b-c, & \text{otherwise} \end{cases} \tag{4.3}$$

The last line works exactly as shown in Eq. (4.1), but the first two were proposed to make the predictor more accurate around the edges. Consider a sharp horizontal edge such as and organ boundary with $c = 0, b = 0, a = 100, p = 101$ (Fig. 4.9). Show that Eq. (4.3) results in lower residual δ compared to Eq. (4.1).

4.11.2   Answers

1. The total size of your data is $S = 100 \times 0.5$ MB $= 50$ MB. If you send it uncompressed, it will take $t_1 = 50$ MB/(10 MB/s) $= 5$ seconds. If you compress it, the data size will drop to $S_{comp} = 50$ MB/$R_c = 50$ MB/3.2 $= 15.6$ MB, which will take only $t_2 = 15.6$ MB/(10 MB/s) $= 1.56$ seconds to transmit. Compression wins? Not at all – don't forget about the 2 seconds to compress and 2 seconds to uncompress this data, changing the total compression scenario time to $t_{2real} = t_2 + 2 + 2 = 5.56$ seconds. That is, the use of the given compression in this case will only delay the image exchange, and uncompressed transmission makes more practical sense.
2. Well, you know that uncompressed image exchange takes $t_1 = 5$ seconds, so we want to transmit everything in $t_2 = 2.5$ seconds. But it takes us at least 4 seconds to compress and uncompress, so regardless of R_c, our compressed image exchange will never be as fast as 2.5 seconds.

   Therefore you need to increase the efficiency of your compression routine, which is the obvious bottleneck in this whole process. You can get a faster processor, or better software implementation (multicore-optimized, for instance). If this will help you drop the compression and uncompression time to 1 second, then you can meet the $t_2 = 2.5$ seconds total assuming $2.5 - 1 - 1 = 0.5$ seconds transmission time. Given 10 MB/s network speed, 0.5 second transmission time corresponds to 5 MB of data, which is one-tenth of your original data size $S = 50$ MB. That is, you can do this with $R_c = 10$.

   Note the difference in factors: tenfold compression yields only twofold faster data transmission. Always do your math before considering the use of image compression.
3. If we use Eq. (4.1), $\delta = a + b - c = 100$. This is a pretty high value because edges make pixels less predictable. However, if we use Eq. (4.3), we must take the second option of $c \leq \min(a,b)$, and our predictor value in this case becomes $\max(a,b) = 100$. That is, Eq. (4.3) yields $\delta = p - \max(a,b) = 1$, which is a much more accurate result. Note that compared to Eqs. (4.1), (4.3) does not introduce any complex computations. So JPEG-LS uses Eq. (4.3) to achieve more accurate predictions around the edges, while keeping computational performance high.

References

Erickson, B. J., Kripinski, E. & Andriole, K. P., 2010. A multicenter observer performance study of 3D JPEG2000 compression of thin-slice CT. *J Digit Imaging*, pp. 639–643.

Fritsch, J. P. & Brennecke, R., 2011. Lossy JPEG compression in quantitative angiography: the role of X-ray quantum noise. *J Digit Imaging*, pp. 516–517.

Golomb, S. W., 1966. Run-length encodings. *IEEE Transactions on Information Theory*, pp. 399–401.

Gulkesen, K. H. et al., 2010. Evaluation of JPEG and JPEG2000 compression algorithms for dermatological images. *J Eur Acad Dermatol Venereol.*, pp. 893–896.

Gupta, N., Swamy, M. N. & Plotkin, E., 2005. Despeckling of Medical Ultrasound Images Using Data and Rate Adaptive Lossy Compression. *IEEE Transactions on Med. Imaging*, 24(6), pp. 743–754.

Kim, K. J. et al., 2011. JPEG2000 2D and 3D Reversible Compressions of Thin-Section Chest CT Images: Improving Compressibility by Increasing Data Redundancy Outside the Body Region. *Radiology*, pp. 271–277.

Kim, T. K. et al., 2012. JPEG2000 compression of CT images used for measuring coronary artery calcification score: assessment of optimal compression threshold. *AJR Am J Roentgenol*, pp. 760–763.

Loose, R. et al., 2009. Kompression digitaler Bilddaten in der Radiologie - Ergebnisse einer Konsensuskonferenz. *Fortschr Röntgenstr*, pp. 32–37.

Peterson, R. C. & Wolffsohn, J. S., 2005. The effect of digital image resolution and compression on anterior eye imaging. *Br J Ophthalmol*, pp. 828–830.

Peterson, P. G. et al., 2012. Extreme Compression for Extreme Conditions: Pilot Study to Identify Optimal Compression of CT Images Using MPEG-4 Video Compression. *J Digit Imaging*, Vol. 25, pp. 764–770.

Pianykh, O. S., 2012. *DICOM: A Practical Introduction and Survival Guide*. Berlin, New York: Springer

Raffy, P. et al., 2006. Computer-aided detection of solid lung nodules in lossy compressed multidetector computed tomography chest exams. *Acad Radiol*, pp. 1994–1203.

Ridley, E. L., 2011. *Lossy image compression affects CAD performance*. [Online] Available at: http://www.auntminnie.com/index.aspx?sec=rca_n&sub=rsna_2011&pag=dis&ItemID=97616

Shiao, Y. H. et al., 2007. Quality of compressed medical images. *J Digit Imaging*, pp. 149–159.

Weinberger, M. J., Seroussi, G. & Sapiro, G., 2000. The LOCO-I lossless image compression algorithm: principles and standardization into JPEG-LS. *IEEE Transactions on Image Procesing*, pp. 1309–1324.

Part II

Making It Better

There is nothing more convolved, obscure, subjective, over-studied and under-used, than medical image enhancement. If I tell you how many days it took me to come up with this sentence, you'll laugh and throw this book away, but... dear ladies and gentlemen of the jury, let me explain myself.

Exhibit one: Open any mainstream PACS workstation, and try to find anything image-enhancing in its user menu. My bet, it won't be easy. The majority of physicians and radiologists do not use image-enhancing filters in their daily routine, for they have no clue of what these filters do, where they can help, and what negative side-effects they might entail. Why bother?

Exhibit two: Open any research-driven medical imaging app, and you will see long lists of "Gaussian", "median", "denoising", "edge-enhancing", "sharpening", "morphological", "nonlinear" and whatever else options. Short-circuited engineering thought has been cooking this technical gumbo for the past half century, vainly trying to thrill clinical minds. And while this homage to thick image-processing bibles was getting only thicker, I've been always wondering who would finally consume the technology apart from the chefs in the kitchen. I do not want to upset you, my fellow engineers, for I am one of your breed, but from the practical point of daily clinical work most of these filters are totally useless. They were not designed to solve any specific clinical problems, their names mean nothing to physicians, and nor do their theories. You can certainly argue that it is not a physician's business to know about the sacred art of pixel transformations– but then please do not expect them to use something they were never meant to understand.

In short, image post-processing (also known as *filtering*) gives us a perfect example of this cognitive abyss, into which many good bits of MI have fallen without even making an echo. What's worse, most of our clinical processes run image-enhancing filters on a regular basis – consider a CT scanner, constantly applying various flavors of raw data reconstruction, filtering and denoising – that we might not even know about. Yet we have to live with their results and consequences.

Apparently, in our wonderful medical profession, not knowing something does not preclude us from using it all the time.

So if you are still laughing, let's laugh together. And since I am catching you in a good mood, let us try to find out – lastly – what all this image-enhancing business is about.

Image Enhancement

5

I am a man of simple tastes easily satisfied with the best

Winston Churchill

Key Points

Once a digital image is acquired, nothing else can be added to it – the image merely keeps the data it has. Nevertheless, different components of this data may have different diagnostic meaning and value. Digital image enhancement techniques can emphasize the diagnostically-important details while suppressing the irrelevant (noise, blur, uneven contrast, motion, and other artifacts).

Physicians don't like image-enhancing functions because they do not trust them. And they have all the reasons to be skeptical. For a good deal of this book we've been playing the same tune: digital data is rigid, and once acquired, it cannot be perfected with more information than it had originally. How, then, can this pixel matrix, so static and invariable, be made any better? Where the enhancements could come from?

The answer is intriguingly simple: they won't come from anywhere. They are already in the image, hidden under the clutter of less important and diagnostically insignificant features. We simply cannot see them, yet they do exist in the deep shades of DICOM pixels. This is why any image enhancement technique – from basic window/level to very elaborate nonlinear filtering – is nothing but an attempt to amplify these most important features while suppressing the least diagnostic. Simply stated, it is sheer improvement of *visibility* of the already present diagnostic content.

This sounds reasonable and easy, but as always, the devil is in the details… To put this puzzle together, we'll do a little case study, departing from the less practical basics, and arriving at something that can actually be used.

5.1 Enemy Number One

Noise is the major enemy of any meaningful image interpretation. Noise is also the most common artifact, inevitably present in every natural object, process, or data – including images. Noise can be purely random (such as "white" noise in X-rays) or

O.S. Pianykh, *Digital Image Quality in Medicine*, Understanding Medical Informatics, DOI 10.1007/978-3-319-01760-0_5, © Springer International Publishing Switzerland 2014

Original pixels p_i ...		
P_1	P_2	P_3
P_4	P_0	P_5
P_6	P_7	P_8

=

...and their sample values		
100	101	100
95	65	97
98	112	103

Fig. 5.1 Small 3×3 pixel sample with noise

more convolved (such as "reconstructed" streak-like noise in CT images) – but if it does not contain diagnostic information, it is useless and destructive. Can it be removed?

Yes, with a certain degree of success, and with a certain artistry of peeling the noise from the noise-free data. To do so, we have to look at it through computer eyes first. Consider Fig. 5.1; it shows a small 3×3 pixel matrix sample with nine pixels p_i, taken from a real image. Do you see noise?

Well, the pixel values p_i are definitely non-constant and fluctuate somewhere around the 100 average. But it is the center pixel $p_0=65$ that really falls out, way too low compared to the surrounding values. Certainly, one may argue that p_0 is depicting some real phenomenon: small blood vessel section, microcalcification, or anything else. But in most cases we expect all diagnostic phenomena to take more than a single pixel (the entire premise behind ever-increasing medical image resolution); one cannot build a sound diagnosis on a single dot. This reasoning brings us to a more "digital" definition of the image noise: abrupt changes in individual pixel values, different from the surrounding pixel distribution.

This means that the only way to remove p_0's noise is to use the neighboring pixels. There are several simple techniques traditionally mentioned when one starts talking about fixing the noisy data. Figure 5.2 shows the most classical one: linear (aka low-pass, Gaussian) smoothing filter. It replaces each pixel p_0 by a new value q_0, computed as a w_i-weighted average of all p_0's neighbors[1] (Eq. 5.1). The positive constants w_i are usually borrowed from bivariate Gaussian distribution:

$$q_0 = \sum_{0 \le i \le 8} w_i p_i,$$
$$w_i = const \ge 0, \quad \sum_{0 \le i \le 8} w_i = 1 \tag{5.1}$$

---

[1] This operation is known as *convolution*: we *convolve* image P with filter W. Note that p_0 is often included into the averaging as well.

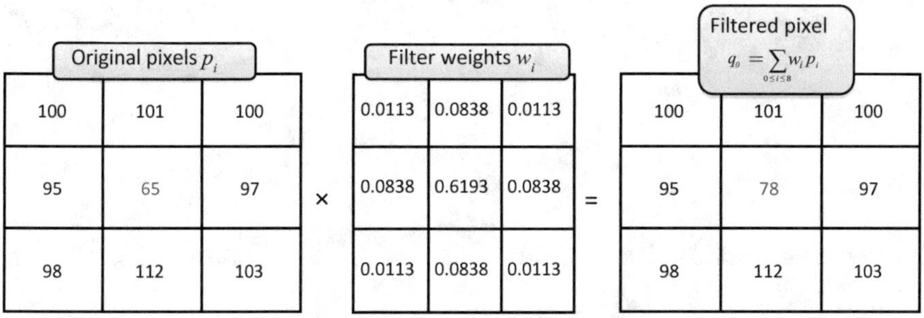

Fig. 5.2 Gaussian denoising. Weights w_i (*center*) were sampled from bivariate Gaussian distribution and normalized to have a unit sum (Eq. 5.1). Summing up p_i values multiplied by their respective w_i produced a filtered pixel value $p_0 = 78$

Averaging is quite simple and intuitive, and if you think about it a bit more, you might realize that it closely relates to both image interpolation (recovering the missing p_0 value with linear interpolation in Eq. (5.1)) and compression (predicting p_0 from its neighbors) – the techniques we discussed in the first part of this book. Yet now we are trying to pitch the same method for removing the noise – should it solve all our problems?

It shouldn't, but in many cases natural noise consists of equally probable negative and positive oscillations jumping around a zero mean. So when we average the pixel values, negative and positive noise instances cancel each other, leaving us with the pure, noise-free pixels. It's reasonable, it's simple, it's easy to compute – in short, it's too good to be true.

Look at Fig. 5.3: averaging leads to smoothing of the image. It reduces the noise at the expense of making the entire image fuzzier.[2] This is why smoothing is useful for extracting large image features, but not for improving diagnostic quality – Gaussian filtering is also commonly referred to as Gaussian blur, and blurring is the last thing we want in image enhancement. This makes Gaussian filters, so abundant in imaging apps, fairly useless for our clinical needs; although good in theory, they fail to provide a decent diagnostic output.

▶ *Nota bene:* The outcomes of imaging filters may be very subtle – can you always spot filter-related artifacts?
   You can, and there are two practical ways to see what you gained and what you lost with any particular filter:
   1. Apply the filter several times. As we learned from the previous sections and Fig. 3.3C, this will accumulate filter artifacts, making them crystal-clear.
   2. Compute a difference image, subtracting original image from the filtered. The difference will show exactly what the image has lost after the filtering.

---

[2] The amount of smoothing depends on the choice of w_i – when they correspond to a sharp Gaussian distribution with small deviation σ, the smoothing will be minimal, but so will be the denoising.

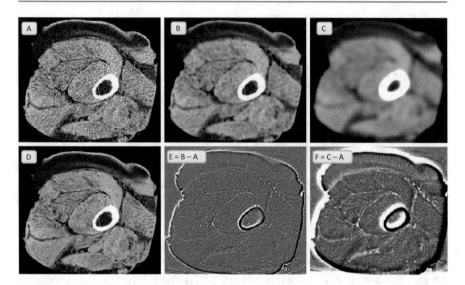

Fig. 5.3 Gaussian denoising filter, applied to the original noisy image A. Image B shows the result of a single Gaussian filtering, and image E shows the difference between B and A. Image C is the result of ten Gaussian iterations (and $F = C - A$) – as you can see, more Gaussian filtering produces even more blur. Image D shows a better original image, initially acquired with less noise. In theory, we want the filtered A to approach D, but Gaussian filtering in B and C loses all sharp image details

We can learn from our little Gaussian fiasco and consider another example of a basic, yet non-Gaussian noise removal approach. Known as a *median filter*, it attempts to fix the blurring problem by using pixel median instead of pixel average:

$$q_0 = \underset{0 \le i \le 8}{\mathrm{median}} \{p_i\} \tag{5.2}$$

– that is, replacing p_0 by the central value from the sorted pixel sequence (Fig. 5.4).[3]

You would probably agree that median-filtered image B in Fig. 5.5 does look better and sharper than its Gaussian-filtered counterpart B in Fig. 5.3. It's true, and median filters can do a pretty decent job removing "salt and pepper" noise – isolated corrupted pixels, surrounded by noise-free neighbors. But this is a rather idealized scenario, hard to find in real clinical data, where neighbors of the noisy pixel will be noisy as well, and so will their medians. Besides, instead of Gaussian blur, the median filter suffers from intensity clustering, exemplified in Fig. 5.5C – when

---

[3] Note that median filter departs from simple averaging just like the JPEG-LS predictive model (shown in the question section of the previous chapter) departs from the basic linear $p = a + b - c$ prediction, for the very same reason: it works better with sharp image details (edges). Many image-processing concepts are intimately connected, and you can often track them in seemingly-unrelated applications, such as denoising and compression in this case.

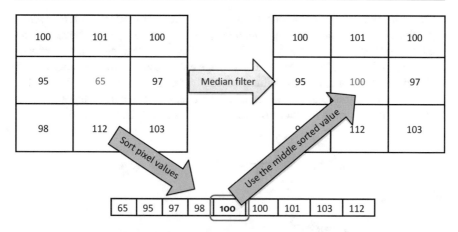

Fig. 5.4 Median filter replaces p_0 with the median value from the $\{p_0,\ldots,p_8\}$ sequence. Medians are less dependent on the outliers, and will not blur the edges

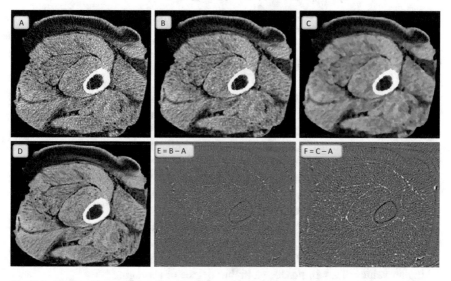

Fig. 5.5 Median filter, and the same imaging experiment: noisy original A, filtered with one (B) and ten (C) passes of the median filter. Image $E = B - A$ and image $F = C - A$. Image D is a noise-free original that we would like to approach with B. Unlike the Gaussian filter, the median filter does not blur, which is why it removes mostly noise and does not touch the structural elements (difference image E shows mostly random noise). However, the median filter tends to grow clusters of same-color pixels – this is somewhat visible in B, and very apparent in C, with its brushstroke-like pattern. This clustering destroys the natural texture of the image, and although we still remove the speckled noise, the filtered images look far from the ideal D

several pixel neighbors start forming same-intensity blobs. This clustering destroys the natural image texture even at a single filter pass – which cannot be accepted in diagnostic denoising.

Nonetheless, the median filter introduces us to the next level of *nonlinear filtering*, which cannot be done with w_i-weighted pixel averaging, used by Gaussian and the like. Nonlinearity proves to be a really fruitful concept, leading to more sophisticated processing, capable of real medical image enhancement. The *bilateral filter* is one of the most popular of the nonlinear breed (Tomasi and Manduchi 1998; Giraldo et al. 2009). To fix the Gaussian approach, the bilateral filter redefines the weights w_i to become non-constant functions of pixel intensities and distances (Eq. 5.3):

$$q_0 = \frac{p_0 + \lambda \sum_{j \neq 0} w_j p_j}{1 + \lambda \sum_{j \neq 0} w_j p_j},$$

$$w_j = e^{-\left(\frac{p_0 - p_j}{\sigma_v}\right)^2} e^{-\left(\frac{\|p_0, p_j\|}{\sigma_d}\right)^2},$$

$$\|p_0, p_j\| = \sqrt{\left(x_{p_0} - x_{p_1}\right)^2 + \left(y_{p_0} - y_{p_1}\right)^2} \tag{5.3}$$

– distance between pixel p_j and center pixel p_0,

$$\lambda, \sigma_v, \sigma_d = const > 0 \qquad \text{– filter parameters}$$

$$e^x = \exp(x) \quad \text{– exponent function}$$

The equation for w_j may look somewhat complex to an unprepared eye, but it has a very simple interpretation: weighting coefficients w_j are made to be high when two pixels p_0 and p_j are close in both location and intensity (Fig. 5.6). In this way, weight w_j defines *pixel similarity*, and neighbors most similar to the central p_0 receive the highest weights. Thus, instead of simply averaging the p_j values with the Gaussian filter, the bilateral filter replaces p_0 with the average of its *most similar neighbors*.

It's easy to understand why this approach can remove noise while being gentler on the local details and edges:

1. If p_0 intensity is significantly different from the surrounding p_j, then w_j will be nearly-equally low, and p_0 will be replaced by an average of its neighborhood. This is the case of the Gaussian filter's removal of a stand-alone noisy pixel; higher values of λ will produce a higher degree of averaging.
2. Otherwise, if p_0 has a few similar pixels around, their weights w_j will prevail in (Eq. 5.3), making the other terms negligible. As a result, the value of p_0 will be adjusted to the average of its most similar neighbors, producing a rather small p_0 change. This is the case of preserving a local image detail, formed by several similar pixels. Thus, the bilateral filter will not make the details fuzzy.

As Fig. 5.7 suggests, bilateral filtering can do a pretty good job in image denoising: it avoids indiscriminate Gaussian blur, and escapes median filter brushstrokes. This makes the bilateral filter a good practical choice for diagnostic image denoising applications, and I would recommend having it on your filter list.

Nevertheless, even the bilateral filter still can be abused and should not be overdone (Fig. 5.7C), and its parameters (λ, σ_v, σ_d) must be chosen wisely to provide the optimal result. Besides, being a Gaussian relative, the bilateral filter will still be smoothing the edge-free areas, where all p_j will have nearly same values, resulting

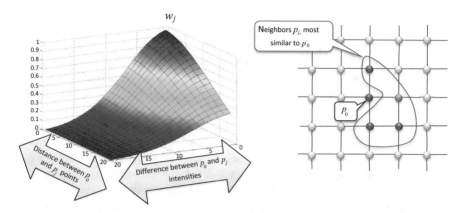

Fig. 5.6 *Left*: Here is how bilateral filter coefficient w_j depends on the proximity between p_0 and p_j, both in pixel intensity and location. When p_0 and p_j become close (differences in their location and intensity approach 0), w_j reaches its maximum, indicating that both pixels are similar and can be used to correct each other's values. Otherwise, w_j becomes negligibly small, meaning that dissimilar p_j should not contribute in the filtered value of p_0. *Right*: The neighbors p_j similar to p_0 will have higher weights w_j, thus contributing more to denoising of the p_0 value

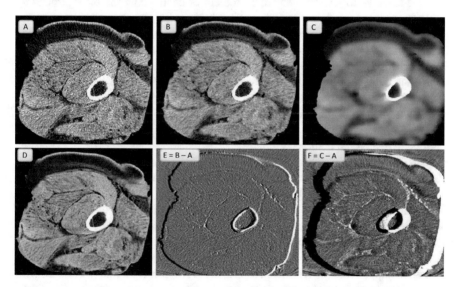

Fig. 5.7 Bilateral filter. In essence, the bilateral filter (single iteration in *B*, and ten iterations in *C*) can be viewed as an "edge-aware" Gaussian: it smoothes only similar pixels. Therefore the result of its application *B* approaches ideal noise-free original *D*. The choice of the filter parameters (λ, σ_v, σ_d) has significant impact on the filtered image quality, and may require preliminary image analysis

in Gaussian-like values of w_j. Eventually, this puts a practical limit on how much noise one can detect and remove by using only the pixel intensity-driven filtering. Therefore more complex image denoising would try to use additional information on how the image was obtained and reconstructed (Choudhury and Tumblin 2003; Balda et al. 2012), but we'll leave this special area outside the scope of this book.

5.2   Denoising Dilemmas

It's good to have a meaningful image-enhancing filter, but it's even better to find the spot where it fits into your clinical imaging pipeline. CT imaging presents an interesting case of practical alternatives, problems and decision-making involved in any clinical image enhancement. Without making a full list, let's consider a few most imperative.

As you might have heard many times, to shoot a sharp CT image, one needs a brighter "X-ray flash" – higher current and a larger number of photons, passing through the patient's body. It certainly makes the pixels perfect, but it irradiates the patients, exposing them to above-average X-ray doses. The radiation that, once it gets in, stays in, potentially contributing to higher cancer risks.

Therefore low-dose CT imagery has been magnetizing clinical minds for a long while. Can we make diagnostic sense of the low-dose CTs? Look at Fig. 5.8: it's a good representation of what happens to CT when the dose goes low – we end up with wild, incoherent noise, coming from the "under-energized" X-ray photons which, instead of passing through the patient's body to make the perfect picture, go astray or get stuck in the denser tissues.

This leads us to a very interesting problem of challenging the old "garbage in, garbage out" axiom: intentionally making low-quality, low-radiation images for patients' safety, but then somehow filtering out the noise to achieve the high-dose image quality. How can we do this, and when should it be done?

Well, this is exactly the question that denoising filters are meant to address, if applied at the right time and place. To begin, let's recall that medical imaging data can exist in two principal formats:

- *Raw data*: the original image format used by the image acquisition method/ device. In essence, these are the measurements performed by the imaging detectors, in detector-specific coordinates.
- *DICOM*: the above measurements converted into a standard digital image matrix. In medicine, this representation comes in the format of a DICOM bitmap, same as we talked about throughout this book.

Going from raw data to DICOM images entails some kind of reconstruction, which in the case of CT means the use of a Radon transform to convert raw CT detector measurements (sinograms) into the lattices of digital pixels.[4] Consequently, noise and any other quality-degrading artifacts will be present in the raw data, and will be remapped into the DICOMs. This leads to two principal image-enhancement alternatives: denoising the raw data, and denoising the reconstructed DICOMs. Which one is better?

Theoretically, raw data denoising would be the perfect approach. First of all, raw data embodies the full volume of the original acquisition – any subsequent reconstructions will drop something out (think about our discussion of digital image interpolation earlier in this book). Second, image noise in the raw data format often

---

[4] http://en.wikipedia.org/wiki/Radon_transform

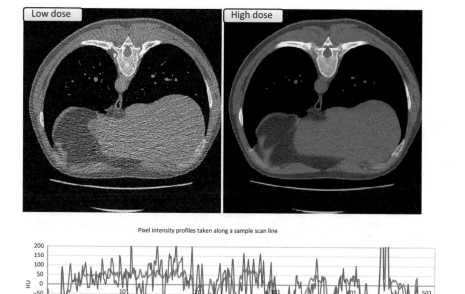

Fig. 5.8 *Top*: Using lower radiation doses in CT imagery results in noisier images (*left*). *Bottom*: Pixel values (measured in CT Hounsfield units, HU) taken along the same line in low- and high-dose versions of the same CT image. You can see how the low-dose pixel values deviate from the much more accurate high-dose measurements

follows the "white noise" pattern, most easily separable from the diagnostic data. And, if we clean the noise from the raw data measurements, we stop it at the very first frontier – before it propagates into DICOM images and everything else based upon them (CAD, 3D, teleradiology, etc.). In short, it would be great, and it is the default way of doing clinical noise removal.

Practically, however, the default may not be the best. First of all, any raw data manipulations are done on the image-acquiring devices, and therefore are nearly always proprietary. It means that different CT scanners will almost certainly run different flavors of CT reconstruction, further complicated by different noise-filtering algorithms. Naturally enough, this will produce images with different, and sometimes incompatible quality (Fig. 5.9). And since these algorithms are built into the scanners, there is nothing you can do to make them better – short of begging your scanner vendors or courting them with exorbitant "software upgrade" fees.[5] Finally, even if you invent a better filtering algorithm, the vendors won't let you run it on their devices.

---

[5] Raw-data denoising algorithms are often offered as optional add-ons, and at quite hefty prices.

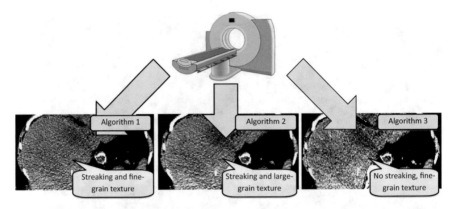

Fig. 5.9 Same CT raw data, reconstructed with three different algorithms. You can see how the choice of reconstruction algorithm affects not only the noise, but also the textural pattern. Diagnostic side-effects of denoising artifacts yet have to be studied

▶ *Nota bene:* The differences in vendor-specific CT filtering may be so obvious (Fig. 3.9), that one can design an algorithm to identify them automatically. Once I was asked to do so, only to discover that images shown in Fig. 3.9 will have very different coefficients in DCT transform – the same transform we mentioned when talking about JPEG compression. So here comes another interesting connection: different reconstruction algorithms affect not only the visual and diagnostic content of the images, but also their compressibility, which in turn affects diagnostic quality of compression-driven projects (such as teleradiology). See how one little alternation leads to a chain of falling dominoes, which we should learn to foresee and to plan for.

Thus, proprietary raw-data filtering can become a true hassle, especially in the typically multi-vendor environments of our hospitals. This convinced many to explore the other alternative – DICOM-based denoising, filtering noise from the reconstructed images wherever they originated. Not only does this provide a vendor-neutral approach to image enhancement, it also enables you to experiment with your own techniques, and to expand denoising to other image types and modalities (X-rays or ultrasound, for instance). With nonlinear filtering, often built on the same concepts as bilateral, one can reduce noise amounts equivalent to 30–50 % of lower CT doses – quite a noticeable improvement for the patient's well-being.

This solves the problem, or does it not? In reality, the DICOM-versus-raw choice of denoising is only the first step in building a sound image-enhancing workflow. Recall how thoughtless compression can make your networking slower, and diagnostic quality – worse. With image enhancement algorithms, you run into the same risks: they take time. Well before the low-dose CT filters of our day, I was visiting the headquarters of a major CT vendor; they had the same filters already, but with one *little problem*: processing a single CT series was taking about 10 h. And although the current denoising has been optimized for much faster results, you should still check its time requirements. This is particularly important for DICOM-based filtering, when you'll need image-processing servers to clean those noisy images before they reach the PACS. To avoid bottlenecking, you'll have to place these servers in well-planned locations, in numbers sufficient to handle your imaging load. To plan for the server throughput, a good rule of thumb would be to use your PACS throughput rates: if you have 15 images/s coming to PACS from the scanners, plan for at least 15 images/s denoising – whatever number of denoising servers it takes. And since numbers translate into dollars, you may end up explaining the denoising post-processing to your CFO – didn't I tell you that medical informatics is fun?

To conclude: practical image enhancement implementation goes well beyond a "Denoise" button pushed in some unknown software interface. Sorry, but you'll have to do the math, and you'll have to do the planning. The good news is that all these alternatives can be weighed *before* you buy a wrong product and start pulling your hair out. Throwing computers at your problems never helps. Thinking and analyzing do.

▶ *Nota bene:* In one of my denoising projects, we used bilateral filtering for DICOM CT denoising, with a target of 30 % dose reduction. To confirm our results and parameter settings, we performed a blind test with radiologists to compare our bilateral-filtered images to the ones obtained with a vendor-specific raw data filtering implementation. To my utmost surprise, both filters were found to be visually and diagnostically identical, equally improving our noisy originals. Who would have thought that DICOM filters, operating with significantly reduced reconstructed data, could rival proprietary raw-data implementations?

5.3   Multi-scale Contrast Enhancement

We spent sufficient time explaining the denoising filters, but…

Do you like music, my dear reader?

Let me assume that you do, whatever your neighbors may think. And whether it's Lacrimosa or The Unforgiven, you might be familiar with the concept of an *equalizer*: rebalancing different frequencies in your digital audio to achieve the most expressive, tailored sound. Believe it or not, but the same concept exists in medical imaging: you can rebalance your images to achieve the best visual quality.

The thing is, noise removal is not the only way to stress the subtle image details. These details may be very hard to see even when noise levels are negligible – simply because those little diagnostic details are overlapped and masked by more massive, but less important, imaging structures. Early signs of pathologies, tiny fractures, little plaques, barely visible tumors can be hidden behind sparse soft tissues, wide bones, and the like. Can we change this unfair imbalance?

We can, if we revisit our earlier noise-filtering experiments. Remember how we got disenchanted with the linear Gaussian denoising (Eq. 5.1) – it was ironing out the little image details, so that many of them were thrown away into the difference image (original minus Gaussian, image E in Fig. 5.3)? Well, this is why Gaussian is known as a *low-frequency* filter (another acoustic analogy) – removing sharp high-frequency details, it leaves us with smoothed low-frequency background. Then, if we subtract the Gaussian from the original… Bingo! – we get the details. This "original minus Gaussian" strategy is called *high-frequency* (aka *unsharp*[6]) filtering, and it opens the door to detail amplification: if we take the high-frequency image (such as image E in Fig. 5.3), amplify it, and add it back to the original, we'll end up with a detail-enhanced image. We show this process in (Eq. 5.4), with pixels equations for the original image P, Gaussian image G, difference image D and sharpened image Q.

$$g_0 = \sum w_i p_i, \text{ (Gaussian } G, \text{ low frequency filter)}$$

$$d_0 = p_0 - g_0, \text{ (detail } D, \text{ original minus Gaussian)}$$

$$q_0 = p_0 + \alpha d_0 = p_0(1+\alpha) - \alpha g_0 = p_0(1+\alpha(1-w_0)) - \alpha \sum_{i \neq 0} w_i p_i =$$

$$= \sum_i u_i p_i \text{ (sharpened } Q, \text{ original plus amplified detail)} \qquad (5.4)$$

where $w_i = const \geq 0, \quad \sum w_i = 1, \quad \alpha > 0,$ and

$$u_i = \begin{cases} 1+\alpha(1-w_0), & i = 0 \\ -\alpha w_i, & i \neq 0 \end{cases}$$

Note that the sharpening filter inherits the linearity of its Gaussian predecessor: sharpened pixels q are obtained from the original pixels p with constant weights u_i (similarly to Fig. 5.2). However, unlike the Gaussian w_i, sharpening weights u_i are no longer positive, which completely changes the outcomes: instead of low-frequency blur, we end up with high-frequency amplification (Fig. 5.10).

Figure 5.10 illustrates the application of Eq. (5.4) to a reasonably low-noise image: the details do become more pronounced. This can already be useful for some of your clinical scans, but it is only a prelude to a more exciting concerto. The real fun begins when we apply (Eq. 5.4) iteratively, rebalancing all available frequency bands. To do so, we send the first Gaussian image G (first line in Eq. (5.4)) down the same pipeline, breaking it into its own Gaussian G_2 (double-Gaussian of the original) and detail D_2 (Fig. 5.11).

This is how we end up with detail images D_n, computed at different frequency levels n – image-processing gurus call this a *Laplacian pyramid*. This is identical to decomposing your music into several frequency bands, just like downsampling is identical to playing in a lower octave. And just like you rebalance your music by amplifying or suppressing its frequency channels, you can rebalance an image by amplifying or suppressing its detail content D_n on different detail levels. Merging

---

[6] Ironically, sharpening filter historically goes under the "unsharp" name.

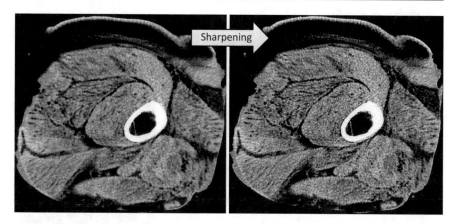

Fig. 5.10 Original (*left*) and sharpened (*right*) images. Beware: sharpening of noisy images will emphasize their noise as well

those amplified or suppressed differences back, we arrive at a frequency-rebalanced image, such as shown in Fig. 5.12.

The Gaussian-based scale decomposition in Eq. (5.1) can be replaced by other decomposition types of the same linear (choice of w_i) or more complex nonlinear nature. Since we lose image resolution at each application of Gaussian, the number of decomposition scales will depend on the image size: the larger the image, the more frequency bands we'll be able to explore. This explains why multi-scale image enhancement has become particularly useful in plain X-rays – such as digital mammography – where you have a large image size on one side, and the need to emphasize small diagnostic details on the other (Laine et al. 1994; Dippel et al. 2002).

This gives us a good example of how the same processing technique (Gaussian) may do very little for one diagnostic task (denoising), and substantially more for another (contrasting) – after a bit of creative "how to" on the processing side, and a bit of better "what to" on the clinical end. This also gives us an example of a truly diagnostically-valuable and meaningful enhancement, which can apply a rather basic formula to produce a pretty impressive result, and which is simple enough to run real-time in a PACS workstation interface. Just as I suggested with bilateral denoising, multi-scale contrast enhancement should be on your shopping list.

5.4   Further and Beyond

Nonlinear bilateral denoising and multi-scale contrast enhancement provide us with two examples of clinically-meaningful image filtering, tuned into solving a particular image quality problem. But the list of these problems is infinite, and image enhancement can go well beyond a basic image cleanup.

To see my point, take any complex image-processing technique, such as 3D, tumor segmentation, or temporal data analysis. When 3D software reconstructs a small artery from a tall stack of CT slices, all it really does is image enhancement – removing

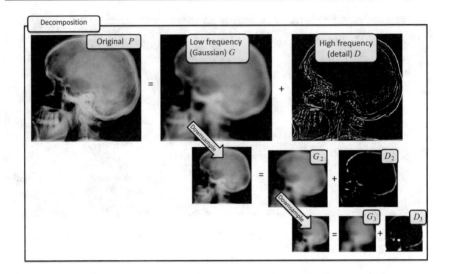

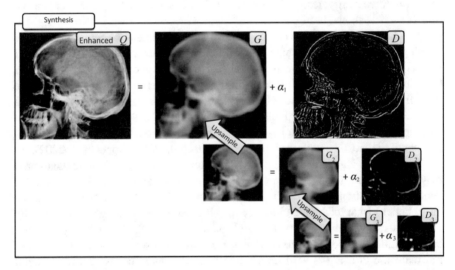

Fig. 5.11 *Decomposition*: Multi-scale image decomposition. At each level, we decompose the image into its low-frequency (Gaussian filter) and high-frequency parts. Since the low-frequency part removes the details (degrades the image resolution) we reduce image size by a factor of 2 (downsample), and then repeat the same decomposition process again. Note how the detail images D_n become increasingly coarser: at each decomposition step, we lower the frequency content of the image, which results in lowering the resolution of its details. The size-shrinking stack of the detail images D_n is known as a *Laplacian pyramid*. *Synthesis*: Reversing the decomposition process. We reconstruct the initial image, but we use detail-amplification coefficients α_n at each decomposition level n. With proper choice of these amplifications, one can arrive at a much better diagnostic image presentation: compare image Q to the original P

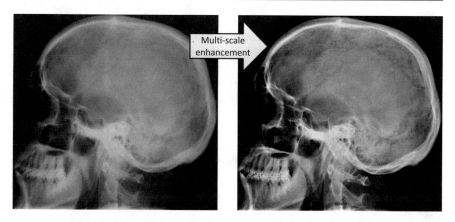

Fig. 5.12 Rebalancing details of the original (*left*) can result in a much improved diagnostic presentation of the same image (*right*)

the least needed, perfecting the most important. In its very essence, image enhancement is the royal road to Computer-Aided Diagnostics (CAD).

This opens several very interesting venues:

- Enhanced images may have very little to do with the originals. Take temporal image analysis (perfusion) as an obvious example. In perfusion processing, one wants to observe the volume and speed of blood flow through various tissues and organs. The originally-acquired images (CT or MR) would somewhat reflect those changes in the varying pixel intensities, but won't let us study and quantify the flow. Therefore we need temporal analysis software to post-process the images, derive the actual blood flow data, and use it to highlight and color the areas of clinical interest, thus significantly enhancing the diagnostic presentation of the original. If interested, you can read about the 3TP method as an example (Furman-Haran and Degani 2002).
- The entire concept of image filtering becomes diagnostically-driven, as it really should be. Running Gaussian or median filters has very minimal diagnostic value, as it serves no diagnostic purpose: these generic filters will suppress the noise (good), but blur or smear the details (bad), so you end up playing a zero-sum game. But once you start looking for something diagnostically-specific (such as an unenhanced tumor), you may want to design a filter to emphasize this particular phenomenon (such as texturing filters – example in Ganeshan et al. (2009, 2012). This is exactly what makes a meaningful interdisciplinary MI project. And it's why, my fellow engineers, we always have to start with the problem, and not with the solution. It's also why, my fellow physicians, we need to know what we are looking for, how to define it, and how to formalize it in the most logical terms – so that we can delegate this job to the algorithms and computers. Instead of doing a monkey's job of randomly pick-

ing blunt weapons from the dusty shelves of math memorabilia, trying to see whether anything fits, we have to work together on designing very precise, razor-sharp algorithms with clear-cut diagnostic purposes.

Bottom line? Analyze. Your image enhancement alternatives can be countless, ranging from extremely simple negative imaging[7] to the most complicated iterative post-processing. Analyze and know what you need before pushing the "filter" button.

5.5   Math: Where Do Good Filters Come From?

"Gee, how do you invent all these filtering equations? Are you just pulling them all from your head?"

Wonderful, wonderful question. Want to know the answer?

No one is making these filters up – they originate from different mathematical concepts, dealing with optimal data properties. Many of these concepts can be viewed in the light of *data regularization*. Regularization means forcing your data to meet certain *regularity criteria*, which you believe the data should satisfy in the ideal, artifact-free case. For instance, the observed, real-life image is always noisy, but the ideal image is pure and noise-free. Can one put "noise-free" into a pixel formula?

Let's try. First, consider our noisy original image P, and its denoised version image Q that we wish to discover. The mean square error between P and Q equals to:

$$E_{or} = \sum_i (p_i - q_i)^2 \qquad (5.5)$$

where p_i and q_i are the corresponding pixel values from the images P and Q. E_{or} shows to what extent Q deviates from the original P, and if you want to find the Q that minimizes E_{or}, you will end up with a trivial result of $Q=P$ ($q_i=p_i$, $E_{or}=0$). The image closest to the original is the original image itself. This is also wonderful, but it does not buy us anything – yet.

We definitely need something less trivial and – knock-knock – here enters the regularization trick. Remember how we wanted Q to be *better* than P, more *regular*? In a good, regular image we expect each pixel q_i to resemble its neighbors q_j of the same type – each organ or tissue should have its proper "birds of a feather" shading. Then we can introduce a measure of inter-pixel similarity as

$$w_{ij} = e^{-\left(\frac{q_i - q_j}{\sigma_v}\right)^2} e^{-\left(\frac{\|q_i, q_j\|}{\sigma_d}\right)^2} \qquad (5.6)$$

---

[7]Robinson and colleagues give a simple illustration of this with a plain grayscale inversion, to improve the visibility of lung nodules (Robinson et al. 2013).

so that w_{ij} are large for pixels q_i and q_j when they are close both in space in intensity (sound familiar?). Then we can define the "irregularity measure" of image Q as follows:

$$E_{reg} = \sum_{j \neq i} w_{ij}(q_i - q_j)^2 \qquad (5.7)$$

Now what happens if we want to minimize E_{reg}? The value of E_{reg} will depend primarily on the terms with the highest w_{ij} – they contribute most to the magnitude of E_{reg}. Therefore, any E_{reg} –minimizing algorithm will target these largest terms first, trying to make their $(q_i - q_j)^2$ factors as low as possible. But high w_{ij} weights correspond to the most similar pairs of (q_i, q_j), correct? Then minimizing E_{reg} will attempt to make those most similar (q_i, q_j) even more alike, moving q_i into its intensity class, defined by the most similar neighbors q_j. That is, minimizing E_{reg} will increase pixel similarity within the same intensity classes (such as specific organs and tissues) – which implies denoising.

If you made it to this point – congratulations, because here comes *la grande finale*: we add E_{or} and E_{reg} into a single error function:

$$E = E_{or} + \lambda E_{reg} = \sum_i \left[(p_i - q_i)^2 + \lambda \sum_{j \neq i} w_{ij}(q_i - q_j)^2 \right] \qquad (5.8)$$

$$\lambda = const > 0$$

With all terms being positive, minimization of E will drive both E_{or} and E_{reg} low and closer to 0. But keeping E_{or} low will ensure that image Q stays close to the original image P, while keeping E_{reg} low will make Q less noisy. In other words, minimal E will correspond to the Q that is a *less noisy approximation to the original* image P (Fig. 5.13). Perfecto! – this is exactly how we wanted to filter the noisy original P. And just in case you enjoyed this mathematical spectacle, note the balancing act played by λ, known as the *regularization parameter*: when λ is small (close to 0), the E_{reg} term is essentially neglected, and minimization of E simply makes Q close to P (minimizes E_{or}). When λ becomes larger, the role of E_{reg} increases by introducing more and more regularization (denoising) at the expense of making Q less similar to P. The optimal choice of λ makes it perfect.

This is really the entire regularization theory in a nutshell, and – let's agree – it is rather intuitive. The only thing that remains is to derive the explicit filtering formula for Q, which can be done by solving Eq. (5.8) for minimum. Due to nonlinear w_{ij} in Eq. (5.6), one cannot solve Eq. (5.8) for q_j directly, so it is usually solved iteratively, assuming w_{ij} constant at each iteration. Under this assumption of temporarily-constant w_{ij} you can differentiate E as a function of q_i. Try it, if you really want to roll your sleeves up – and you will arrive (surprise!) at the bilateral filter formula in Eq. (5.3). In other words, the famous bilateral filter is nothing but a regularization solution, obtained from Eq. (5.8)! Quod erat demonstrandum.

Certainly, math may not be something that makes you shiver with joy, but the purpose of this little exercise was hardly to entangle you in a web of confusing

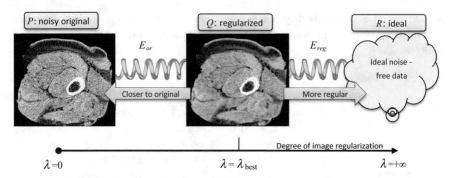

Fig. 5.13 Regularization allows us to settle the denoised image Q between the original noisy P and our idealized image representation R (not even an image in itself). As always, the truth is in the middle, and this is where we converge by choosing the most appropriate λ

formulas. What is really important is to understand that image-enhancing filters have a very solid and logical foundation, and do not come from random jangling with obscure code. On the contrary, they spin off from the fundamental concepts of making imperfect real data more consistent, which is what regularity really means. They also open the gates for countless experiments and improvements, because anything from filtering parameters (such as $\lambda, \sigma_v, \sigma_d$) to regularity functions (such as E_{reg}) can be defined in many interesting ways, depending on what you expect from the ideal data (Choudhury and Tumblin 2003). Math merely gives you the tools –the thinking still should be all yours.

5.6   Self-check

5.6.1   Questions

1. Why must the sum of w_j in Eq. (5.1) be equal to 1?
2. Show that Eq. (5.4) generalizes to Eq. (5.1).
3. What image enhancements would benefit your clinical practice? How would you implement them?

5.6.2   Answers

1. This is how we ensure that the average image intensity remains the same. To see this for yourself, assume that all p_j are equal to some p. Then

$$q_0 = \sum_{0 \le i \le 8} w_i p_i = \sum_{0 \le i \le 8} w_i p = p \sum_{0 \le i \le 8} w_i = p .$$

That is, if all p_j (p_0 included) had the same intensity, this intensity will be preserved -by filtering. This makes perfect sense: same-intensity areas should remain intact; they have nothing to filter out.
2. Hint: consider $\alpha = -1$.
3. It's *your* practice. Think!

References

Balda, M., Hornegger, J. & Heismann, B., 2012. Ray Contribution Masks for Structure Adaptive Sinogram Filtering. *IEEE Transactions on Medical Imaging*, pp. 1228–1239.

Choudhury, P. & Tumblin, J., 2003. The Trilateral Filter for High Contrast Images and Meshes. *Eurographics Symposium on Rendering*, pp. 1–11.

Dippel, S., Stahl, M., Wiemker, R. & Blaffert, T., 2002. Multiscale Contrast Enhancement for Radiographies: Laplacian Pyramid Versus Fast Wavelet Transform. *IEEE Transactions on Med. Imaging*, 21(4), pp. 343–353.

Furman-Haran, E. & Degani, H., 2002. Parametric Analysis of Breast MRI. *Journal of Computer Assisted Tomography*, pp. 376–386.

Ganeshan, B., Miles, K.A., Young, R.C. & Chatwin, C.R., 2009. Texture analysis in non-contrast enhanced CT: Impact of malignancy on texture in apparently disease-free areas of the liver. *European Journal of Radiology*, pp. 101–110.

Ganeshan, B. et al., 2012. Tumour heterogeneity in non-small cell lung carcinoma assessed by CT texture analysis: a potential marker of survival. *European Radiology*, 22(4), pp. 796–802.

Giraldo, J. et al., 2009. Comparative Study of Two Image Space Noise Reduction Methods for Computed Tomography: Bilateral Filter and Nonlocal Means. *Minneapolis, IEEE EMBS*.

Laine, A.F., Schuler, S., Fan, J. & Huda, W., 1994. Mammographic Feature Enhancement by Multiscale Analysis. *IEEE Transactions on Med. Imaging*, 13(4), pp. 725–740.

Tomasi, C. & Manduchi, R., 1998. Bilateral Filtering for Gray and Color Images. *Bombay, IEEE International Conference on Computer Vision*, pp. 839–846.

Robinson, L.W. et al., 2013. Grey-scale inversion improves detection of lung nodules. *Br J Radiol*, 86(1021), pp. 1–5.

Image Quality Online

6

To prepare asparagus, you will need to rinse the
spears and break off the tough ends.
After that, how you cook asparagus is up to you.

Online recipe for cooking asparagus.

Key Points

With web-based imaging getting increasingly widespread, we should become more aware of its quality-specific aspects. Running diagnostic imaging in a web browser, on a limited-bandwidth public network will almost certainly affect the original image quality. Online image-viewing applications must know how to compromise between the speed of image access and the preservation of original image depth and resolution. They should also provide cross-platform and cross-browser compatibility, and intelligent management of their limited resources.

If you happen to be in medical imaging for some time, you might recall those wonderful scholastic battles of the 1990s: can computer monitors provide the same diagnostic display quality as printed film? As with anything else asked from your IT department, the original answer was "No", or rather "No!!!", multiplied by the imperfections of the early computer monitors, and raised to the power of notorious clinical conservatism. And while most kept printing and arguing, others preferred to invest the intervening years in perfecting the digital display technology – eventually winning the market and the dispute. Oh those acid-smelling printing monsters of the old days… "Where are the snows of yesteryear?"[1]

Nonetheless, history likes to repeat itself, and the same question "is new always evil?" was resurrected a few years ago, this time with online image viewing versus then-abhorred and now praised PACS monitors. The correct answer was already known – "we will get online sooner or later". And while the most conservative of us laughed at the dubious reports of "Look, I can read CTs on my cell phone!" reports (undoubtedly dissipated by the fifth column of IT-poisoned renegades, shattering the medieval piers of our clinical science), the most creative of us did the same job – they took web display and browser technology to a qualitatively new level. First ActiveX, then Java, and now new and enhanced JavaScript provided for efficient

---

[1] François Villon.

O.S. Pianykh, *Digital Image Quality in Medicine*, Understanding Medical Informatics,
DOI 10.1007/978-3-319-01760-0_6, © Springer International Publishing Switzerland 2014

and function-rich diagnostic browsing. Display technology made its quantum leap to the point when resolution and brightness of portable gadgets started to rival those of old and bulky PACS monitors. Network bandwidth (enhanced by compression and network protocol fine-tuning – see impressive results in Langer et al. (2011)) approached real-time distribution benchmarks.

Problem solved?

At the basic, fundamental web-viewing level – yes. These days, wisely-designed, thoughtfully-balanced web applications can deliver nearly native image viewing experience; you will not feel much "remoteness". But the first successes only opened the gates for more tempting advances, and more rigorous improvements. Let's look at some of them, most related to the image quality subject of this book.

6.1   Finding the "Web" in Web-PACS

The terms "web-PACS" and "cloud-PACS" have become very trite these days, and radiologists keep discussing different online systems as something they've known for ages. But when you start following these discussions, you will suddenly see different groups of people talking about totally different things. Web-PACS, very much like teleradiology, is often understood in the most liberal sense of remote PACS connectivity. If I run a PACS workstation on my PC at home, loading my hospital images, I have a web-PACS, right? Or don't I?

I do not. This is a standard PACS setup, as we have known it since the mid-1990s. Doing imaging from a remote location does not make it "web". So let's be a bit more careful with our definitions. A true web-PACS means a PACS client, which can run in a web browser (Internet Explorer, Safari, Chrome, Mozilla,…) and

• Does not require installation: the users open it as they would open any web page
• Does not leave any context information or data after it shuts down – no "footprints", essential for protecting data confidentiality[2]
• Can be invoked from a third-party application through its URL[3]
• Balances functionality between itself (client) and its backend (server). For example, the server may be fully DICOM-compliant, while the web client would be merely doing the image presentation part.

In this case, the entire World Wide Web becomes your image-viewing environment, where full server-based PACS should transform itself into a web service.

As natural as it looks, this design took a while to develop. The first standalone PACS were not "web" at all, although they already used networks to exchange their

---

[2] This is the most common requirement in what is known as REST architecture. REST stands for REpresentational State Transfer; read more at http://en.wikipedia.org/wiki/Representational_state_transfer

[3] So a link like http://MeWebPACSServer?PatName=JoeSmith&PatID=123456, entered by hand or generated by another third-party application, will launch the web viewer with Joe Smith's images already loaded into it.

data. Neither were emails with low-res JPEG attachments, FTP files servers or shared folders, and (no, please, do not do this again!) remote desktop connections to PACS workstations. All these "innovations" made an awesome pile of insane projects and pointless presentations, but kept all us walking backwards until, by the late 1990s, it was realized that common sense cannot be abused indefinitely, and that web-based PACS should have something far better to offer.

At first, the vendors chose the path of least resistance (surprise!) by simply embedding their bulky systems into browsers with ActiveX-like components. In plain language this meant that a PACS viewer could be started and run from a bowser, but had to be installed anyway, very much like a stand-alone application. Although it was a very little step forward, it was still a totally faked approach to web, contradicting nearly all points on our list above. So by early 2000, the most adventurous companies started exploring Java as a much better web-viewing platform. Java would run on top of Java Virtual Machine (JVM) – special Java-processing code, embedded into each web browser. Users could freely download and install JVMs from www.java.com, instantaneously making their browsers Java-aware and beefed-up for serious image processing. Java's "Write once, use anywhere" motto, supplemented by complex processing functionality, sounded really promising.

However, the entire Java cross-platform promise was based on assumed JVM consistency, while each major software player was trying to develop its own JVM. That sounded like a big trouble from the very beginning, and that's exactly what it turned out to be. As Java grew more and more complex, its JVM implementations started to diverge[4]; their vendors started to argue (famous Sun vs. Microsoft lawsuit); and their users started feeling the pain. In short, the aura of great and powerful coffee-bean technology has shrunk, and its attractiveness for the web PACS implementations has lost most of its gleam (Fig. 6.1).

Fortunately enough, by the time of the early 2000s a much better client-server paradigm finally started to make its way into the clinical applications. Sure, ActiveX or Java were powerful enough to handle full DICOM in web clients, but this same power made them too heavy-weight and complex, and too platform-specific to be used universally. The client-server model was taking a different approach: all heavy processing and standardization were left to the server, and all plain viewing – to the client (hence the *thin* client nickname). From our point of view, it solved two fundamental problems:

1. Complex DICOM- and image-processing functionality was removed from the clients, making their code much lighter and efficient.
2. As a result, lighter, *thinner* clients were less-demanding on the browser side. "Less-demanding" in functionality always translates into "more universal" in implementation: simpler things are easier to run in different browser platforms (Fig. 6.2).

---

[4] Making the ironic "Write Once, Debug Everywhere" a new Java slogan.

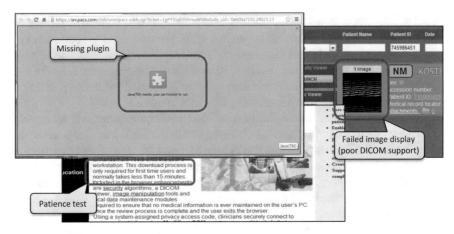

Fig. 6.1 Dealing with plugins has become one of the most upsetting problems in web-based medical imaging – when you need to see your images online, you may not have the patience to wait for "less than 15 minutes" or to deal with non-responsive. Besides, when limited plugin functionality met with DICOM image complexity, failures were common, and resulted in impossible to view images

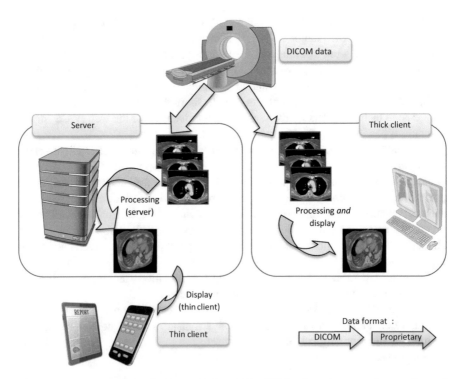

Fig. 6.2 Two concepts of web clients, thick and thin. Thick clients do most of processing and therefore require full original data and complex processing code, which makes them dependent on the particular implementation platform and web browser. Thin clients (used in contemporary web PACS) are used mostly to display the information already processed on the server, so that they are easily supported by a wider range of devices

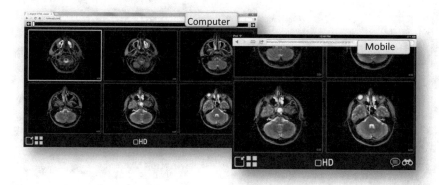

Fig. 6.3 Screenshots of the same thin web-PACS client (www.itelerad.com), taken from PC (*left*) and iPad (*right*) screens. Despite different platforms and browsers (IE vs. Chrome here), the client provides nearly-identical viewing experience regardless of the underlying device. Note the "HD" button, provided to show the images in their original resolution

The new server-client architecture revived the long-misfortunate concept of universal, cross-browser web-PACS: web servers started to do all the work, relieving web clients from massive plugins and imaging code. For that reason, plain HTML with JavaScript – the ubiquitous browsing functionality supported on all platforms, mobile devices included – proved to be absolutely sufficient on the client side, and web-PACS implementations in their true sense started to flourish, becoming a de-facto industry standard. Newly-released HTML5, with its new functionality and image-aware *canvas* object, already supported by major web browsers, only boosted the advances of lightweight clinical imaging (Fig. 6.3).

How has all this affected image quality?

- First of all, with a few minor exceptions, thin clients do not do DICOM. It is not their business. Therefore what you see on a thin client display might be a JPEG screenshot[5] of the true image from the server. Consequently, everything we said earlier about JPEG and lossy compression artifacts applies to web-PACS viewing: beware of lossy imaging!

- Streaming compression might be present in some web clients, although it is getting less and less popular due to the changing image quality experience it produces – unbearable for most doctors.

- Image resolution can often be sacrificed to keep the images smaller for fast client-server uploads. Therefore our earlier discussion on image interpolation applies as well: zooming into the low-res images will produce all interpolation artifacts discussed earlier. To support the original image quality, web-PACS clients will also use the same old trick with low resolution for interactive imaging

---

[5] Lossy JPEG is used more frequently as it is natively supported by all web browsers – which is not the case for JPEG2000 and other advanced compression algorithms. Nevertheless, a good diagnostic thin client should always have a lossless compression option.

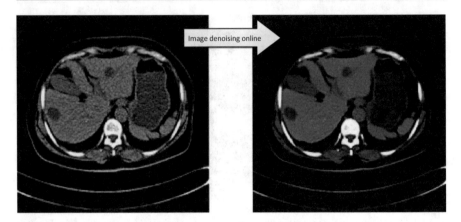

Fig. 6.4 Denoising CT low-dose images online with HTML5 (Hao et al. 2012). *Left*: original noisy low-dose image. *Right*: same image with noise removed

(such as fast scrolling through an image sequence), and original high resolution for diagnostic viewing (once the interactive part is over).

- Thin clients' displays come in all shapes and varieties, and change constantly. This affects the entire paradigm of DICOM calibration – adjusting display brightness distribution to make as many shades visible as possible. In the old times of local PACS monitors, DICOM calibration was easily enforced with regular monitor calibrations, performed with calibration photometers and software. This is not possible with smartphones – therefore better calibration approaches are desperately needed. We will discuss this later in the book.
- Web has become the first place where "I want my images fast" collided with "I want my images best!" This has never been the case with the local PACS, and it polarized the MI audience. In many emergency situations, the "fast" argument may win over the "best" one (Peterson et al. 2012); image quality has lost its omnipotence.

On the other side, web imaging has increased the reach of diagnostic quality, providing it to areas and under conditions where it was not available before (think about the entire teleradiology field). Moreover, the sheer toolset of online medical imaging has been expanding to new and more challenging functions. Consider the recent advances in HTML5, which gave raise to previously unthought-of online image processing – such as web-based CT image denoising (Hao et al. 2012) (Fig. 6.4). I mentioned the new canvas object in HTML5 – it provides access to the image pixels on the client side, re-enabling thin clients to improve diagnostic image quality and presentation.

As web technology becomes more and more complex, we certainly do not want to fall into the old Java trap – when the "thin" became thicker, and the "sophisticated" eventually degraded into the "inconsistent", impossible to support and painful to write. And this is exactly the place where client-server architecture should guard web-PACS from client-specific implementations: servers must remain the common denominators of their web apps. When several instances of the same web-PACS are launched from the same server, they are guaranteed to be consistent, as their functions are coming from the same server box. When we move more functions into clients running on different devices, we risk reopening Pandora's "write once, debug everywhere" box.

6.2   Gadget Radiology

The experimental approach, the cornerstone of medicine, sits on a very practical principle: use what is available to use; ignore the ideal. As we mentioned earlier, this is what makes medicine so much different from the perfectionist approaches of the pure math, hidden behind any informatics application. And the proliferation of gadgets in modern medicine supports the same practical point: consumer tablet computers may be hard to carry around, they may suffer from spills and falls, they may not have convenient medical interfaces, they may not be running the right algorithms or have enough processing power – but they are definitely everywhere. In fact, the notion of making an ideal clinical tablet[6] seems to be overshadowed by the pure prevalence of non-clinical tablets.

Therefore with the same practicality in mind, the question of "Can I read diagnostic images from my gadget?" had been addressed countless times in countless clinical experiments. The question obviously falls into two:

- Can the gadget of choice provide the image viewing specs sufficient for medical imaging? After several years of techy advances the answer has settled on "yes": resolution, brightness, and contrast of current mobile computers easily match the viewing guidelines for most imaging modalities.
- Can the gadget-viewing experience provide enough comfort and efficiency for productive diagnostic work?

The second question is very subjective and is therefore harder to answer, which is why many clinical groups experimented with gadget-versus-workstation comparisons. Abboud et al. (2013) found no significant differences in interpreting chest tuberculosis images on iPad, compared to a standard PACS workstation (Table 6.1).

A similar study carried out by the Imperial College Healthcare National Health Service (NHS) Trust in the U.K. confirmed that, with the exception of CT pulmonary angiograms, reading emergency CT cases on an iPad did not have statistically significantly higher overall error rates compared with reading these cases on PACS workstations[7] (Table 6.2). In emergency workflow however, the use of tablet computers provided much faster 24/7 access to the images, which was considered a major improvement.

These observations were echoed by many similar experiments, which would take another book to enumerate: the time when the quality of your images was thought

---

[6] Such as Motion C5t from www.motioncomputing.com

[7] www.auntminnie.com/index.aspx?sec=rca&sub=rsna_2011&pag=dis&ItemID=97689

Table 6.1 iPad performing nearly identical to PACS workstation for tuberculosis (TB) readings, as reported in Abboud et al. (2013). Two hundred and forty chest images were reviewed by five independent radiologists on both PACS LCD monitors and iPads; each case was graded as TB-positive or TB-negative. The numbers in bold red show the only two cases of disagreement

		iPad	
TB reading agreement		Positive	Negative
Workstation	Positive	38	1
	Negative	1	200

Table 6.2 Typical iPad error rates observed by NHS

CT exam type	iPad
Abdomen	Major: 0 % Minor: 20 %
Head	Major: 3 % Minor: 17 %
Kidney, ureters, and bladder	Major: 0 % Minor: 8 %
Pulmonary angiogram	Major: 27 % Minor: 13 %
Cervical spine	Major: 0 % Minor: 16 %
Overall	Major: 11 % (vs. 6 % on PACS workstations)
	Minor: 37 % (vs. 20 % on PACS workstations)

to be proportional to the weight of your workstation has long passed. In fact, the only weak point for the wild range of mobile gadgets was total lack of a consistent approach to their DICOM calibration; i.e., making their monitors show image intensities in the best possible way for our vision system. We will return to this matter later in the book.

6.3   Web Development: What Should I Consider When Buying/Designing a Diagnostic Web Viewer?

It is always interesting to peek under the hood and see what this web viewing is all about. If you are an MD, you may read this section for the benefit of your software shopping. If you are in IT, you can use this for your development and implementation needs.

First, we are talking diagnostic imaging; therefore, whether it's web or not, the right choice of imaging format is a must. Alas, our trusty DICOM, conceived in the late 1980s, entered this world way before the omnipresent WWW and browsers; it was never meant to work with them, it was never meant to fit into them, it was not even meant to go anywhere beyond the fixed point-to-point connection between two static IP addresses (Pianykh 2012). Recent DICOM extensions (WADO,[8] MINT[9])

---

[8] Part 18 of DICOM standard, ftp://medical.nema.org/medical/dicom/2006/06_18pu.pdf

[9] Medical Imaging Network Transport, https://code.google.com/p/medical-imaging-network-transport/

were developed to address this problem, but they are still far from widespread, and may not answer all of your implementation questions. This leaves you with the two choices mentioned earlier:

- *Thick client*: Designing and implementing a 100 % DICOM-compatible browser plugin.
- *Thin client*: Using a client–server approach, where DICOM images are processed on the server, and displayed in the thin client in some other image format.

The first option may sound very exciting – having DICOM standardization and DICOM image quality all the way through the web would be great – but it's also the least practical. First of all, DICOM is not easy: with all its parts, chapters, encoding types, compression algorithms, image formats, pixel conversions, and proprietary tweaks it may take megabytes of code to implement, at least if you want to have it clean (don't you?). This will turn your plugin into a big fat monstrosity, taking time to download, power to run, and nerves to manage. To overcome all these problems, you will almost certainly have to narrow your viewer down to a specific platform or browser, which in WWW world would be a huge step back. Besides, it may not be worth the effort: your web client does not need to behave as a fully-compliant DICOM application (DICOM "application entity"), because most DICOM functions, handshakes and protocols would be a waste in the web viewing case. Have I convinced you? – stay with the second option.

The second option, however, is not decision-free either, as you will have to ponder over the best image format for the web client imaging. As we've mentioned, many will be tempted to use JPEG, but as we know by now, it is really the worst possible choice: browser-compliant JPEG is not only lossy, it's also 8-bit per grayscale pixel, while DICOM needs up to 16 bits. With all human ingenuity, you won't be able to squeeze DICOM pixels into JPEGs without breaking the diagnostic image quality. The only imaginary way to avoid this problem would be to split the DICOM image into several JPEGs, covering different ranges of DICOM intensities – JPEG to show DICOM bones, JPEG to show DICOM soft tissues, JPEG to show lungs, JPEG to show livers, etc. But hey, this is really just what it sounds like – a dead end; manipulating this pile of JPEGs would be a challenge in itself, likely killing the rest of your app.

All this means that you need to pick an image format that can natively handle up to 16 bits of diagnostic DICOM imagery. This brings us to another pair of options:

- *Using proprietary image format*. Your server can take the original DICOM, do all the dirty work, and repackage it into some "simplified DICOM" of your own design, easy enough to be opened in a thin client.
- *Using well-known image format*. There are image formats that can handle 16 bits per pixel – take PNG or JPEG2000 as example – and your server can convert DICOMs to them for web viewing.

Many vendors go with the first option, but it has one little problem: you still need a plugin to decode your proprietary "simple DICOM". Therefore it is much more efficient to stay with the format that any web browser can understand by default, which is our option number two. JPEG2000 would be the best, as it offers both lossless and lossy compression, which you can use to adapt to the varying network speed – but unfortunately JPEG2000 support in web browsers is practically non-existent. So when we were working on our web viewer, we picked PNG: it can hold DICOM pixels without any degradation (diagnostic quality requirement), and it can do lossless compression (faster download requirement), with absolutely no plugins required. The only downside of PNG is that it does not have a lossy compression option, which would have been so appreciated on slower connections (smartphones). But if you are a developer, you may think about creating a lossy PNG extension, by slightly altering the pixel values to make them more PNG-compressible (see the first part of this book). Done on the server, it will still convert DICOM into the standard PNG, but with higher compression ratios.

▶ *Nota bene:* The easiest way to implement a lossy PNG would be to round image pixel values p to the multiples of some integer K; K = 2 or K = 4, for example:

$$p' = K \times \text{round}\big((p + K/2)/K\big)$$

- This will degrade the image quality (as any lossy compression would do anyway), but when compressed with the standard PNG:Higher K will result in higher PNG compression ratio R_c.
- With this roundoff approach, you'll know exactly that your pixel value was changed by K/2 units at most, which makes it very similar to the diagnostic compression approach used by JPEG-LS ($\varepsilon = K/2$), discussed previously.

Another obvious way would be reducing the image resolution, although it is less desirable: as we already know, the quality loss will be more significant, plus you will have to deal with all resolution-dependent parameters, such as DICOM pixel size in millimeters, which you'll have to update accordingly.

By now I think you should be getting the full sense of this project: even seemingly obvious decisions such as online image format are not as simple as they might sound at first. If you are shopping for the web viewer, talking to several vendors, ask them the same questions we just addressed, and see whether they can come up with a plausible story. The answers "you won't see the difference anyway" should never count; as we should realize by now, the only way not to see something is to guarantee that it cannot be seen. In other words, the only way to provide diagnostic image quality in a web viewer is to guarantee that it is provided by the proper choice of the imaging format – it's that "simple".

Enough? Hey, we just got it started, barely scratched the surface, and it may take another book to go through all web-viewing intricacies. But let's check a few more, just to feel the full range of the problems that a good diagnostic web viewer is expected to solve.

Say we decided to use PNG as our online image format. How would this affect the functionality of the viewer?

In the server-client architecture we've chosen to use, both server and client can perform certain functions, but anything complex and time-consuming should be done on the server, while everything light and fast belongs to the thin client. Take the *Window/Level* (W/L) function – image contrast and brightness adjustment, so frequently used by radiologists.[10] Do we keep it on the server, or do we implement it on the thin client?

Well, let's think. Doing it on the server would be certainly easy – when the user wants to change the contrast and brightness of the image, the client only needs to capture the new W/L value, send it to the server, have the server update the image, and send the updated image back to the client. Simple, but... wait a second, does it mean that we'll have to send back and forth every image we want to update?

It sure does, turning the simplest W/L into a massive internet traffic bottleneck. It will definitely work great on a fast network and an idle server, but have you seen those in reality? I have not, and in web development I wouldn't recommend counting on the ideal scenarios. Moreover, most physicians are used to adjusting image contrast interactively – dragging a mouse over the image and seeing its contrast change instantaneously, proportionally to the smallest mouse displacement. This simply won't fly in the server mode. Hence, it needs to be done on the client.

But doing W/L implies changing the displayed pixel values: brightness adjustment shifts pixel values by some offset, and contrast multiplies them by some factor. Therefore your web client needs to use a technology that can scale and offset image pixels. You cannot do it with a simple HTML – the language just does not have the brains for the pixel processing. This is precisely why, until recently, Java has been the most practical choice: providing full control over the image pixels, Java enabled web developers to manipulate pixels on the client side, without countless trips to the server.[11] Moreover, Java was virtually the only choice for developing functional cross-platform web viewers, had it not run into the problems we outlined earlier. Fortunately enough, as Java struggled, much lighter JavaScript matured enough to provide its own pixel-manipulating and plugin-free mechanism. Some new, better technologies may emerge by the time you open this book, but just stop for a second here and think, how peremptorily one single W/L function shaped most of your web viewer design.

▶ *Nota bene:* Note that W/L solves another important problem, quintessential for web imaging: it allows us to show 16-bit DICOMs on plain 8-bit monitors of our PCs, tablets and smartphones. Without that functionality, we would have remained tied to those bulky "hospital grade" radiological monitors. Thank you, W/L!

---

[10] We'll discuss W/L more in the final part of this book.

[11] I'd like you to note this very important thing, which we touched upon in passing: with web viewing in particular, the choice of functionality may completely define the choice of implementation. This is why it's so hard to improve an ill-designed web viewer: it may be easier to rewrite it from scratch, changing the underlying implementation.

W/L is only a single example; image quality will and should affect all parts of the diagnostic web viewer design. Image volume would be another illustration of the same point. Before the WWW times, images were stored on the local computer hard drive, to be opened and displayed as needed. This was the most efficient way, but as the sizes and lengths of scanned sequences continued to skyrocket, even stand-alone PACS workstations began to stumble over the multi-thousand image stacks.

But guess what? In web viewing, we don't even have the luxury of the local hard drive! First, the hard drive may not be available for security reasons (many web apps will be banned from accessing local hard drives); second, it may not be large enough anyway (think about smartphones). This changes the entire image-viewing paradigm – without large disk storage, where would you put some 2000 CT slices from a cardiac study you need to look at? Where would you keep those enormous angiography cine loops that take hundreds of megabytes to store?

▶ *Nota bene:* Interestingly enough, the lack of a local hard drive is another reason for not using DICOM in the web client. In the standard DICOM networking, the images are commonly loaded by studies or by series – DICOM has no concept of prefetching the "next few images" on demand. Therefore, if you have to view a series of 1000 CTs with DICOM, you are pretty much bound to load them at once – which will most certainly lead to a big browser kaboom, after a few minutes of freezing and waiting. On the contrary, thin clients can be programmed to pick and fetch the images selectively, avoiding the whole-study image overload.

Not using local disk storage created an interesting "side-effect" known as "zero footprint" viewing: when you close the web viewer, it leaves no imaging or patient data on the local machine. Vendors love advertising this as a great security feature, but it is really a byproduct of the same disk-free web architecture. Nonetheless, it's a rare example of a good side-effect, which enables you to view the images from public computers without worrying about your patient's privacy.

The only answer to the no-disk architecture is caching the images in the computer memory – or more precisely, the memory that this particular browser can allocate to the viewer for handling its data. This memory will be far more limited than the good old hard drives, and the only practical way of using it would be fetching the images on demand, instead of loading them at once. To do so, the web viewer will usually start with some low-quality thumbnail-like previews, just to give you a rough idea of what you are looking at. The previews won't be diagnostic (unless you are looking for a broken leg), but they won't take much of this precious memory, and will help you scroll to the slice you are interested in. Once you get there, you will have the option to reload the same slice in full diagnostic quality: either by clicking on some "Full quality" button, or letting the viewer do it by default. Some viewers try to be more intelligent by fetching full-quality versions of a few images before and after the current one, just in case you want to explore the adjacent slices. But "more intelligent" means higher memory overflow risks, and may be done only if the client has good control over the browser memory – you don't want to run into any memory problems.[12]

For the same reason, when you scroll to the new image location, the previous high-quality images will be dropped from the memory to make room for the new ones. Therefore, when you return to the first viewing spot, the high-quality slices will have to be reloaded again, which takes some time. This is the point where many would get really upset: "I just looked at this slice a minute ago, and now I have to wait for it again?" True, but this is the price you are paying for the luxury and convenience of online diagnostic viewing.

Finally – and probably most importantly if you are shopping for a diagnostic web viewer – you must not neglect the matter of cross-browser and cross-platform implementations. Let's face it: having "Internet Explorer only", or worse, "Internet Explorer 9 only" web viewer is a joke, degrading the entire concept of a freely-available WWW. The same applies to the viewing platforms: the era of "PC vs. Mac" battles ended long time ago. Now you have to deal with a slew of computers, netbooks, smartphones and tablets, running all possible flavors of operating systems that human ingenuity and coding lameness have produced over the past decade.[13] Moreover, the outcomes of browser and computer wars change every month, and depend on the region and country – you just cannot bet on any particular *product*, so you absolutely have to build your web viewing on a *technology*. But even the most widespread technology turns into a challenge when you are looking for "cross-everything" implementations: just like with any standard (DICOM is a perfect example), HTML or JavaScript will have countless proprietary deviations specific to each browser or platform. It does not mean that you cannot have it clean; but it does mean that you'll have to work on *making it clean*.

Bottom line? When shopping for a diagnostic web viewer, try to test it on your smartphone, and ask your colleagues to do the same. Moreover, if you want to have real practical fun, test it on your eBook reader – you won't see the best images, but you should see the viewer pages work (Fig. 6.5). One picture will tell you much more than a thousand words from the vendor's advertisement.

---

[12] Some web viewers are smart enough to sense the size of the browser memory, so they know how many high-quality images can be prefetched.

[13] Never underestimate the inertia of hospital IT departments, which just love to run systems several years behind the market. The dinosaur computers you might find in the hospital's "Jurassic Parks" may be extinct anywhere else.

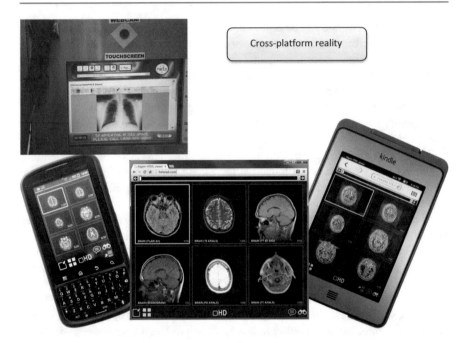

Fig. 6.5 At different times, the author of this book was involved in various web-imaging application development efforts. A long time ago, we started with Java, running diagnostic imaging on virtually everything, including web-enabled payphones (shown on *top* – remember those?). Now one can definitely develop a robust cross-platform viewer to run on smartphones, computers, tablets and even eBook readers (bottom row: same viewer, different platforms). Sure, the latter have terrible image quality, but this is a hardware issue; the viewing application should and can run flawlessly, regardless of the underlying platform and software

6.4   Self-check

6.4.1   Questions

1. Name a few limitations of web-based image viewing.
2. Name some advantages of web-based image viewing.
3. Consider a complex image processing algorithm – such as temporal perfusion analysis, for instance – that your hospital wants to make available on all physicians' smartphones. Should the solution be server-based or client-based? Why?

6.4.2   Answers

1. You may come up with a longer list, but here are some considerations: limited functionality (Javascript and Java won't let you implement the full range of functions available in stand-alone applications); limited memory (web app memory

will be constrained by that of the browser); limited access to the local hard-drive, if any (typical security limitation for web apps); lack of standardization (medical imaging standards like DICOM do not work well with the WWW, although some extensions are being developed).

2. What we gain most of all is universal, installation-free access to the imaging data. If done properly, the web display will run in cross-browser, cross-platform mode, untying you from particular operating systems or devices. Zero-footprint will help you overcome security problems: web apps do not store anything on the local disk, and once you shut them down, you can rest assured that no confidential patient data will remain on the host computer. And with all this, we can still achieve diagnostic quality – not bad at all.

3. This definitely calls for a server-based setup, where all complex processing will be done on the server, and smartphones will simply be displaying the processed data (i.e., acting as thin clients). There is no way you can do the entire processing on the client, smartphone side: limited smartphone memory and processing power, and gazillions of possible smartphone models, make this impossible to implement and maintain. Process on the server, convert to a simple screenshot, display on smartphones.

References

Abboud, S., Weiss, F., Siegel, E. & Jeudy, J., 2013. TB or Not TB: Interreader and Intrareader Variability in Screening Diagnosis on an iPad versus a Traditional Display. *Journal of the American College of Radiology,* pp. 42–44.

Hao, L. et al., 2012. *Enhancing low-dose CT images in the EHR based on HTML5.* s.l., s.n., pp. 97–100.

Langer, S. G., French, T. & Segovis, C., 2011. TCP/IP Optimization over Wide Area Networks: Implications for Teleradiology. *J Digit Imaging,* pp. 314–321.

Peterson, P. G. et al., 2012. Extreme Compression for Extreme Conditions: Pilot Study to Identify Optimal Compression of CT Images Using MPEG-4 Video Compression. *J Digit Imaging,* 25, pp. 764–770.

Pianykh, O. S., 2012. *DICOM: A Practical Introduction and Survival Guide.* Berlin, New York: Springer.

Part III

What You See Is What You Get

"I have seen my death!"
Frau Roentgen on seeing the first X-ray of her hand.

Images come to us through our eyes. This may sound remarkably trivial, but it's remarkably important as well. Our *Human Visual System* (HVS) is a very complex beast, with its own peculiar taste and a very unique sense of humor. Quite often, even the most professional training in medical image interpretation cannot break the magic crystal of HVS deception. Quite often, what we see does not even exist (Fig. III.1).

But we got used to it, and certainly wouldn't care about the HVS tricks, were they not embroiled in the complex mix of diagnostic imaging. Can we see the real images? Can we compensate for illusory distortions? Moreover, can we use HVS to our advantage?

Let's try to answer some of these questions.

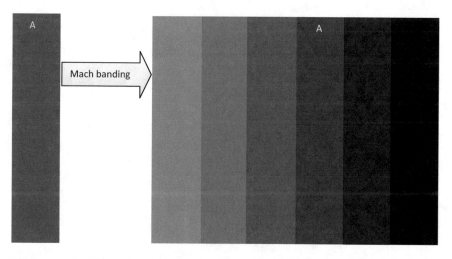

Fig. III.1 Objectivity challenge. One of many tricks HVS plays on us is *Mach banding*. Each grayscale strip on this image has constant intensity – you can easily verify this by checking any of them separately (see strip A on the *left*). But when you see them together, the left side of each strip seems to be *darker*, and the *right – brighter*. This artifact is completely imaginary, yet we perceive it as entirely real

Image Display

7

Key Points

The range of medical image intensities typically exceeds that of commercial displays. This creates a need for various intensity transformations, from plain contrast/brightness enhancements to complex nonlinear intensity rebalancing, which can help explore the rich contents of imaging data.

It is not about what you look at, it's all about what you *see*. From this point of view, an acquired image is nothing but a huge dataset, which still needs to be fed to your visual sensors, transmitted to your neurons, and processed with the latest version of your brain's firmware. No wonder we need to repackage the imaging data so that it reaches our brains in the most meaningful way. This section will help us understand the mechanics of repackaging.

7.1   From Window/Level to Gamma

Let me assume, my dear reader, that you are somewhat familiar with the concept of *Window/Level* (W/L), briefly mentioned before. Also known as brightness/contrast adjustment,[1] W/L helps us zoom into various ranges of image intensities that typically correspond to different tissues and organs. You can find W/L in virtually any medical imaging application, not to mention the remote control of your TV set.

W/L has one important property: it is linear. This means that it maps a selected subrange of the original image intensities $[i_0, i_1]$ into the full $[0, M]$ range of display luminance, using a straight-line function (Fig. 7.1). That's what makes it so similar to zoom: in essence, W/L magnifies all $[i_0, i_1]$ intensities by a constant $\dfrac{M}{i_1 - i_1}$ factor, so that they can span the entire range of monitor luminance. All intensities below i_0 are truncated to 0, and above i_1 – to M.

---

[1] Or "contrast enhancement", "contrast stretching", "intensity stretching" etc.

O.S. Pianykh, *Digital Image Quality in Medicine*, Understanding Medical Informatics, DOI 10.1007/978-3-319-01760-0_7, © Springer International Publishing Switzerland 2014

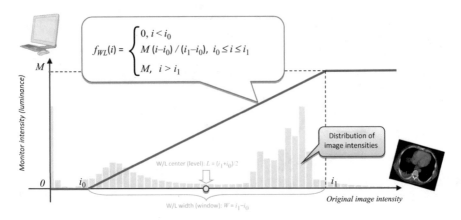

Fig. 7.1 Window/Level function displays a selected range of the original image intensities $[i_0, i_1]$

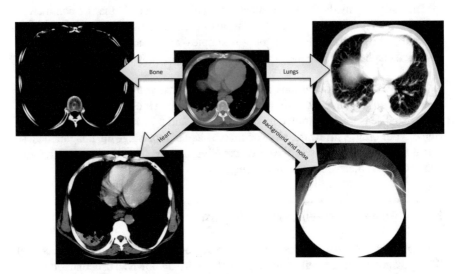

Fig. 7.2 Use of linear W/L transform to select different $[i_0, i_1]$ intensity ranges in CT image. Note that the image includes everything from diagnostic tissues to pure noise

W/L is probably the most frequently used button on your diagnostic workstation toolbar, and it does a wonderful job of localizing different organs and tissues (Fig. 7.2). W/L is also the only practical way to explore the full intensity spectrum of 16-bit DICOM images, using that plain 8-bit monitor sitting on your desktop. As we pointed out earlier, 16-bit medical images can contain up to $2^{16} = 65,536$ shades of gray, while plain consumer monitors can show only $2^8 = 256$ of them at once. Clearly, 65,536 does not fit into 256, but W/L solves this problem, enabling us to browse through the original 65,536 shades, displaying only the intensities that matter to us at any particular moment – such as $[i_0, i_1]$ range in Fig. 7.1. Without W/L,

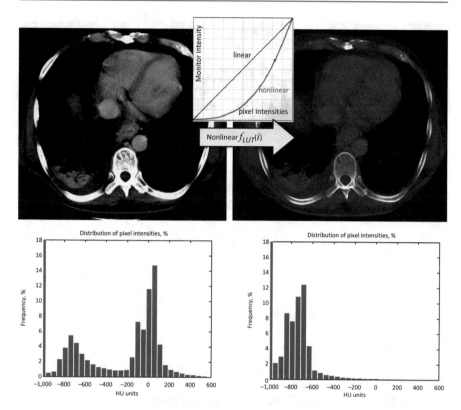

Fig. 7.3 Nonlinear intensity transformation. Unlike W/L, which merely selects intensity subranges, nonlinear transforms change the distribution of pixel intensities. The graphs under the images show their histograms – plots of pixel value frequencies. Note how bright intensities centered around zero HU on the *left* histogram disappeared – they were moved into the darker intensity ranges of negative HUs

we would have to depend on more complex and considerably more expensive monitor hardware capable of displaying deeper than 8-bit grayscale – hardware that may be hard to find and install. In essence, it was the W/L function that contributed to the proliferation of teleradiology, smartphones, tablets and web viewers, to reach far beyond the grasp of your bulky PACS workstation.

In short, we should all bow and thank W/L for being so useful and handy. But you, my inquisitive reader, would certainly like to go beyond the basics, wouldn't you? So what if we consider nonlinear, curved mapping? Look at Fig. 7.3: unlike the "bone" example in Fig. 7.2, this transform improves the original bone contrast, but you can still see the soft tissues. This suggests a nonlinear function $f_{LUT}(i)$, which cannot be expressed as a fixed-factor intensity zoom. Instead, it amplifies different intensities with different factors – less for darker, and more for brighter. If we want to keep our zoom analogy, this is similar to the fish eye effect.

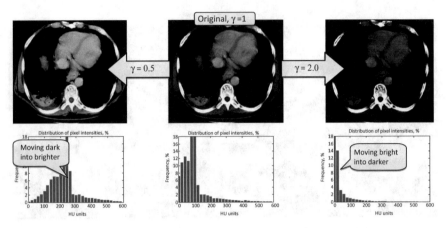

Fig. 7.4 Gamma correction, applied to the [0, 600] range of the original pixel values (expressed in CT HU units)

For example, consider $f_{LUT}(i) = f_\gamma(i) = M\left(\dfrac{i}{i_{max}}\right)^\gamma$ for some constant value $\gamma > 0$. This power transform is known as *gamma correction*. When $\gamma = 1$, it is linear $f_{\gamma=1}(i) = i\dfrac{M}{i_{max}}$, which is identical to a W/L transform with $W = 2 \times L = i_{max}$. However, the more different γ becomes from 1, the more nonlinearly $f_\gamma(i)$ behaves – check out Fig. 7.4, which illustrates the differences in $f_\gamma(i)$ for $\gamma = 0.5$ Wnd $\gamma = 2.0$. You can see that $f_{\gamma=0.5}(i)$ amplifies lower (darker) intensities at the expense of suppressing the higher (brighter) ones. Therefore for $0 < \gamma < 1$, it is often called "dark enhancement", as it improves the visibility (contrast) for the dark image shades. For the same reason, $\gamma > 1$ provides "bright enhancement".

What is particularly interesting is that the "dark vs. bright" rebalancing helps gamma correction to undo some of the HVS artifacts. Our visual system works better in the dark: humans see more contrast in dark shades than they do in bright ones. This helped our little furry prehistoric ancestors hunt and survive at night. For that reason, if we want to see as objectively as digital cameras and medical scanners do, we need to compensate for this "night-day" nonuniformity. This can be done if we pack more image shades into the dark part of the luminance spectrum – the part where we can see better, and therefore can see more. But this is exactly what gamma correction does for $\gamma > 1$ – it moves more image shades into the darker luminance spectrum (Fig. 7.4, right). Thus, we arrive at our first attempt to achieve HVS-neutral image display, with nothing but a simple $\gamma > 1$ power transform.

This ability to make shades more visible is one of the reasons that gamma correction became popular with graphics hardware manufacturers. Many displays would be preconfigured to use γ around 2.2 to make the images more vivid – that is, packing more shades into our favorite dark-intensity zone. This luminance arrangement also enables us to differentiate among more similar shades. Make a mental note here – we will revisit the "more shades" approach and magic $\gamma > 1$ a bit later, when we talk about DICOM calibration.

Finally, from the implementation point of view, nonlinear intensity transforms lead to an interesting concept of *Look-Up Tables* (LUT) – a concept that profoundly affects the ways we look at the images. The problem is that nonlinear functions like $f_{LUT}(i)$ can be quite complex. In fact, they may not even have easy formula-like expressions. Recomputing $f_{LUT}(i)$ every time and for every pixel would simply kill any image-processing application. This is why the simplest way to store and apply nonlinear transforms is to keep them in tables: for each original image intensity i we define the corresponding display luminance $m_i = f_{LUT}(i)$. Then once m_i are stored in the LUT, we read them from there instead of recomputing $f_{LUT}(i)$ values again. Think about using some LUT transform while scrolling through a long stack of MR images: every pixel in every image will have to be transformed with $f_{LUT}()$ before it is thrown on the screen. This is exactly the case when calling $f_{LUT}()$ for all pixels will take forever, but fetching $m_i = f_{LUT}(i)$ from the LUT table – a few instants.

▶ *Nota bene:* Without a doubt, you can also use LUT to tabulate the linear W/L function $f_{WL}(i)$. But when it comes to hardware implementation, linear transforms can usually be defined and applied directly, without the need for any LUT; besides, not using LUT saves memory. Complex nonlinear transforms, on the contrary, need LUT format to be stored in computer memory. This does imply certain memory overhead, but we do not have to compute complex transform values every time we need them. Thus, we gain performance.

7.2   Histogram Equalization

Gamma correction is a good but still quite basic example of pixel intensity remapping. *Histogram Equalization* (HEq) is another yet more complex example of improving image perceptibility. It does a really interesting job of making all image shades *equally visible*.

Let's look at Fig. 7.5. The original image has only a few active shades: a massive dark background (hiding lots of low-intensity details) and a cluster of bright colors. So its histogram – the distribution of pixel intensities – is extremely unbalanced (Fig. 7.5, left distribution). This makes you wonder whether it makes sense to support those 65,536 medical grayscales if only a few shades do the real job. A bit wasteful, isn't it?

Well, we can try to improve the dark shades with $0 < \gamma < 1$ gamma correction – say, by using $\gamma = 0.5$. It does make the dark more visible (Fig. 7.4, left), but it would not be able to fill the unused intensity gaps. On the contrary, we would like to spread out all intensity levels as equally as possible, to make them all stand out.

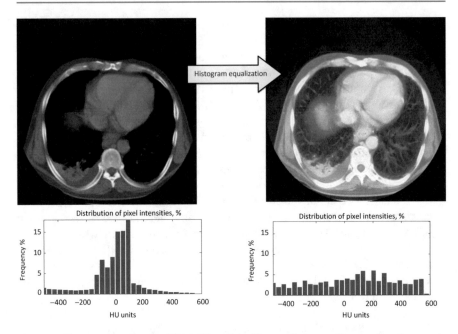

Fig. 7.5 Histogram equalization (HEq). The original image histogram (frequencies of grayscale pixel values) looks very unbalanced; HEq makes all frequencies nearly equally probable

Histogram equalization was designed to solve this very problem by redistributing the shades more uniformly over the entire image intensity spectrum. Here is how it works. Consider a grayscale image with pixel intensities i_n taking values from 1 to N. Let's assume that each intensity level $i_n = n$ occurs c_n times. Then, if C is the total count of all image pixels, we find $\alpha_n = c_n/C$, the probability of pixel intensity (shade) $i_n = n$. Consequently, cumulative probability $A_n = \sum_{k=1}^{n} \alpha_n$ gives us the fraction of all intensities with value n or less.

If all intensities in the image were equiprobable, we would have

$$\alpha'_n = 1/N$$
$$A'_n = n/N \qquad (7.1)$$
$$n = NA'_n = i'_n$$

The intensities in a real medical image won't be distributed uniformly, and Eq. (7.1) won't hold true. Moreover, we cannot do anything about the intensity probabilities α_n either – for instance, if a background color of $i_0 = 0$ can be found in $c_n = 1,000$ pixels, we cannot "split" $i_0 = 0$ into several different shades. But we can use the last line in Eq. (7.1) to redefine the intensity values a bit better. That is, to approach the uniform distribution of pixel intensities, we can remap the original $i_n = n$ into new intensities j_n such that

$$j_n = f_{HEq}(i_n) = NA_n = N\sum_{k=1}^{n} \alpha_n \qquad (7.2)$$

Given c_n and N of the original image, we compute α_n, and we define and j_n according to Eq. (7.2), rounding all j_n to the nearest integer values. This will redistribute the original intensities over the entire $[1,N]$ intensity range in the most uniform way.

As Fig. 7.5 (right) demonstrates, the result may be quite impressive. All of a sudden you can see a whole lot more: soft tissues, bones, lungs, even the clothing around the patient's body. In fact, in most instances HEq images will look way too busy because they render virtually all image details in a single view. But this is why HEq can be so handy: it can uncover hidden structures and expose subtle details, simply invisible otherwise. If you are looking for anything hidden, it is worth checking the HEq images; you may learn something from them.

▶ *Nota bene:* In the basic histogram equalization described here, we used pixel intensity as the only pixel property. If we consider other local pixel features – such as the average intensity of the pixel neighborhood – we can arrive at more elaborate equalization approaches, with even better differentiation among close shades. If you are interested, I recommend reading (Coltuc et al. 2006). Note that more complex equalization techniques, which depend on more than single pixel intensity, will have to be implemented as pixel-processing filters, and not as intensity LUTs.

Histogram equalization gives us a good example of image-specific LUT, which has to be derived from the intensity distribution of a particular image. It's also a good example of the intensity transform $f_{LUT}(i) = f_{HEq}(i)$ not having a simple formula; as we have just seen, histogram equalization requires probabilistic image analysis, which definitely takes some time to process. Therefore it is exactly the case when we want to compute the equalized $f_{HEq}(i)$ values once, and then store them in a LUT memory, to be used as many times as needed without incurring new processing costs. This example shows us that LUTs can be used in two principal ways:

1. LUTs can be applied to selected images, based on specific image properties. This is how HEq works: it depends on the image, therefore each image will need its own HEq LUT. For that reason, image-dependent LUTs require software implementation.
2. LUTs can be applied consistently to all displayed images, regardless of their properties. Gamma LUT is a perfect example: it does not need to know anything about the original image intensities and their distribution. Such image-independent LUTs can be implemented directly with display drivers and hardware.

Although both scenarios call for different implementation approaches, they still spring from the same LUT idea of "compute once, use many times".

7.2.1 Colorization

One of the few LUT applications you'll find in virtually any medical imaging software would be colorization. There is a good reason for this. The majority of medical images are grayscale: they display the amplitude of a particular imaging signal, such as electromagnetic fields in MR and CT, or sound waves in ultrasound. This response, being one-dimensional by definition, naturally maps into a one-dimensional grayscale. Alas, there are no other dimensions to color the picture.

But our visual system can certainly recognize colors, and colors can transmit extra information about the objects. This points us to the idea of artificial *colorization* – or *color mapping* – to enhance the diagnostic presentation of grayscale originals. Colorization is usually done for one of two reasons:

1. To highlight additional imaging phenomena: temporal changes, dual energy, varying degrees of pathology, etc. This implies specific image processing and computer-aided diagnosis so it cannot be accomplished with a simple LUT approach (see interesting examples in Wiemker et al. (2012) and Kim et al. (2009)). Therefore we will leave this topic for another investigation.

2. To improve image presentation: consistently mapping the original grayscale image pixels into color display pixels. This can be definitely done with LUTs, often referred to as "palettes" or "color ramps".

Figure 7.6 shows an example of color mapping – and you will probably agree that the colorized versions might give you more cues about the subtle changes in tissue shading. The most popular color ramps found in virtually any medical imaging software would be spectral, thermal, hot, and cold (Fig. 7.6). These palettes look great but.... they have no clinical meaning. Their connection to the original data is completely random, and their color range may depend on the current intensity window (images C and D in Fig. 7.6). As a result, what is red on one image may end up being green or blue on another. Worse, artificial colorization can induce artificial color boundaries, when several very different hues may fall on the same organ (see purple, green and blue indicated by the arrow in Fig. 7.6C). This disconnect creates an illusion of changed tissues, distorting the real organ continuity (Rogowitz et al. 1996).

▶ *Nota bene:* A few years ago we were installing our new PACS software in a hospital, replacing an aging product from another vendor. Everything worked well until we suddenly received an ultimatum from the radiologists reading plain X-rays. They refused to use our program on one single ground: it did not have an option for spectral X-ray colorization, available in the previous product. The radiologists kept insisting that it would help them see fractures.
Luckily we were able to implement the LUT, and the problem was solved. But the lesson was learned as well: in medicine, what seems superficial to some might be essential to others.

With so many potential problems, the only advantage of artificial colorization lies in its ability to make subtle details more visible. Some physicians find it useful, and some argue against (Tofangchiha et al. 2012). Therefore, to find a more solid approach to color mapping, we need to ask ourselves what colors we are expecting

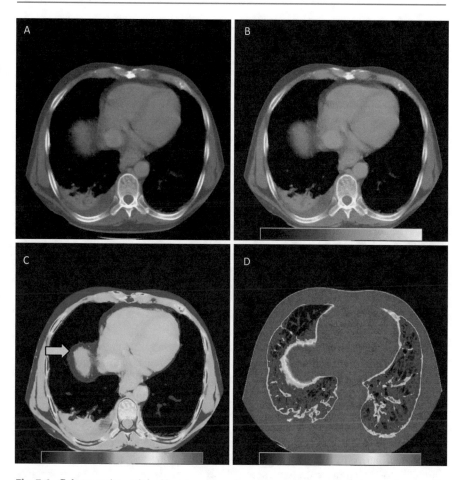

Fig. 7.6 Color mapping: original image *a*, thermal ramp *b*, spectral ramp *c* and spectral ramp with changed W/L window *d*. Although *c* and *d* use the same color map (strip at the *bottom*), the map is applied to different ranges of the original image intensities, producing entirely different colorization

to see. The most typical answer is the natural, anatomical colors of human organs and tissues. *Realistic coloring* can help us highlight true abnormalities, which makes it handy in many areas, from surgical planning to teaching. But can it be achieved if we have nothing but grayscale to begin with?

The short answer is "No":

- Our grayscale pixels may not have any absolute units, or any relationship to the natural organ colorization; consider MR imaging with various choices of acquisition protocols. The colors we see belong to the visual spectrum, different from what most imaging modalities use.

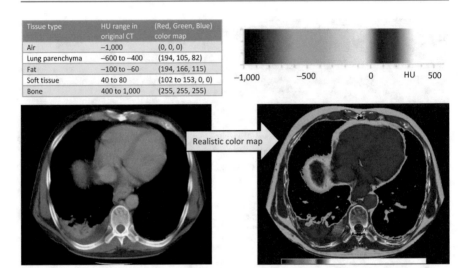

Tissue type	HU range in original CT	(Red, Green, Blue) color map
Air	−1,000	(0, 0, 0)
Lung parenchyma	−600 to −400	(194, 105, 82)
Fat	−100 to −60	(194, 166, 115)
Soft tissue	40 to 80	(102 to 153, 0, 0)
Bone	400 to 1,000	(255, 255, 255)

Fig. 7.7 Realistic CT color map proposed by Silverstein et al. (2008) and its application in CT colorization

- Even when grayscales are clinically consistent – such as Hounsfield densities in CT imaging– the problem of realistic colorization has no straightforward solution: the same CT grayscales can correspond to very different organs, without any clear-cut connection to the anatomic organ coloring. In other words, you cannot tell from a black-and-white photo of an apple whether the real apple was green, red, or anything in between.

Nonetheless, one can still try to suggest an approximate colorizing LUT, comparing real anatomy images (from surgery and from projects such as Visible Human[2]) to their grayscale equivalents. This comparison can lead to reasonably good colorization, especially when it is limited to particular organs and image acquisition protocols. This pragmatic approach was applied by several researchers (Silverstein et al. 2008), with one of the examples illustrated in Fig. 7.7.

Thus, if you're thinking about colorizing your grayscale data, ask yourself first *what* your colors should mean. Whatever answer you have, it should be rooted in the intrinsic properties of your data values, and not in some unscrupulous "let's make it prettier" approach. Finally, bear in mind that the HVS response to colors is even more complex[3] – there are countless color artifacts, problems with the same colors perceived differently at different luminances, or by different viewers. Therefore, even color images may need their own color calibrations – such as calibration of human wound photographs described in (Van Poucke et al. 2010).

---

[2] http://www.nlm.nih.gov/research/visible/visible_human.html

[3] CIELAB standard models HVS color perception, http://en.wikipedia.org/wiki/Lab_color_space

The more colorization connects to the objective properties of your data, the better it will be.

▶ *Nota bene:* Vision is our principal imaging tool, but the most creative of us have experimented with the other human senses. For example, audible prompts and hints are often used in visual interfaces to enhance our image perception. Browse the Web, and you will find software to convert images into sounds – try this to improve your diagnostic reading!

7.3   Local W/L: From LUTs to Filters

Standard linear W/L works great and keeps many happy, but it has one problem: once you zoom into that specific $[i_0, i_1]$ intensity range, you cannot see anything outside of it. For example, if you use a CT "bone" window (looking at bone density range), you lose soft tissues, and vice versa. Wouldn't it be nice to see everything at once?

Well, you can guess that it is impossible to window/level all image densities at once – you simply won't be able to squeeze an arbitrary number of image intensities into a limited number of display luminances M. But here is an idea: what if we break the original image into a mesh of small squares (8×8 pixels, for instance), and do W/L for each of them, optimally mapping each square's intensity into the entire $[0, M]$ luminance range of the monitor?

This is exactly how local (nonlinear) W/L works (Fig. 7.8) – it applies optimal contrast stretching to each small fragment of the original image. In a sense, this is somewhat similar to histogram equalization, but now your goal is to provide the *optimal contrast* in *each* pixel neighborhood. The result is also similar to that of HEq – you see much more in a single image. Yet, unlike redefining grayscales on the global scale with HEq, local W/L preserves tissue structure around each pixel, while considerably improving the visibility of the whole. This is why local W/L can be used to compensate for uneven organ densities, such as breast density in mammography. After local W/L, the organ looks as if it was equally flat, revealing the structures otherwise hidden behind the denser parts.

Can you do local W/L with a single LUT transform, like everything else we've studied so far? Definitely not; as Fig. 7.8 suggests, in the case of the local W/L we need a separate intensity map per each little neighborhood square. That is, we need a lot of little local LUTs, or a LUT that depends not only on the image pixel intensities, but on the pixel locations as well. This is where we depart from the basic LUT concept, leaving it for another occasion. But this is exactly the place where simple LUTs are superseded by image filtering, discussed in the second part of this book, and this relationship needs to be understood and appreciated. Just like image postprocessing filters are trying to emphasize the diagnostic content of the images, LUTs are trying to make this content as visible to our eyes as possible. This is how these two virtually unrelated concepts meet each other, and even overlap in the case of local W/L – a centaur looking half-LUT, half-filter. Interesting, isn't it?

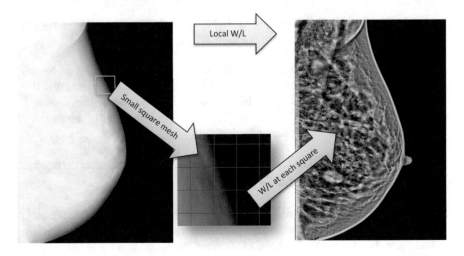

Fig. 7.8 Local W/L transform applied to compensate for breast thickness

7.4   Self-check

7.4.1   Questions

1. Can we use LUT to implement image denoising?
2. Can LUT transform be undone?
3. Consider a conventional color monitor: it has 16 million colors, but only 256 of them are grayscales. Can we somehow use the monitor colors to simulate deeper grayscale imaging?

   This is not an easy problem, but it has at least one elegant solution. To find it, think about another interesting feature of our human visual system: we can differentiate intensities much better than colors.

7.4.2   Answers

1. No. The entire point of LUT is to consistently map each image intensity i into a corresponding display intensity $m_i = f_{LUT}(i)$. With denoising, pixel value i can be corrected (denoised) differently in different locations; it may be replaced by m_1 in one spot, and by m_2 in another. LUTs cannot do this.
2. Definitely, unless you saved the modified pixels instead of the original. Practically, any LUT can be implemented in two ways: using display hardware (if it can support this particular LUT transform), or modifying image pixel values. If you use the hardware approach (such as contrast or gamma adjustment, likely available in your monitor settings), the original image is not touched, and returning to the original settings will undo the transform. But in most cases the transform has to

be implemented in the application itself. In this case, novice software developers simply keep applying LUTs to the same image, remapping its pixels into the new values – unfortunately, this destroys the original data and we cannot go back to it unless we reload the image again from its file. The correct approach is to keep two images: the original, and the one used for display. Then we can use any LUT to transform the original image into its display version, but we still keep the original. Undoing LUT then amounts to resetting the display copy to the original image.

3. Our eyes are much more sensitive to overall pixel intensity than they are to hues. This phenomenon can be used to trick our vision into seeing more grayscales than technically possible. In the classical (R,G,B) color space, the gray shades will correspond to the integer (R,G,B) triplets with $R = G = B$: (0,0,0), (1,1,1),...,(255,255,255). Now consider two consecutive grayscales like $g_{100} = (100,100,100)$ and $g_{101} = (101,101,101)$. In theory, we cannot add anything else between them. But what if we add two more slightly-colored shades like $a_{101} = (100,100,\mathbf{101})$ and $b_{101} = (100,\mathbf{101},\mathbf{101})$?

The color hues in a_{101} and b_{101} are so minor that your eyes won't see them. Yet the intensities of a_{101} and b_{101} will be somewhere between g_{100} and g_{101} – slightly brighter than g_{100}, and a bit darker than g_{101}. And this is what we were looking for: with minor, unperceivable colorization we just added two more shades per each original grayscale, thus increasing our perceived grayscale count to $256*3 = 768$. Sometimes we can fool our own visual system to our advantage!

References

Coltuc, D., Bolon, P. & Chassery, J.M., 2006. Exact histogram specification. *IEEE Trans Image Process*, pp. 1143–1152.

Kim, K.W. et al., 2009. Quantitative CT color mapping of the arterial enhancement fraction of the liver to detect hepatocellular carcinoma. *Radiology*, pp. 425–434.

Rogowitz, B.E., Treinish, L.A. & Bryson, S., 1996. How not to lie with visualization. *Com Ph.*, pp. 268–273.

Silverstein, J., Parsad, N.M. & Tsirline, V., 2008. Automatic perceptual color map generation for realistic volume visualization. *J Biomed Inform*, pp. 927–935.

Tofangchiha, M. et al., 2012. Detection of vertical root fractures using digitally enhanced images: reverse-contrast and colorization. *Dent Traumatol*, pp. 1–5.

Van Poucke, S. et al., 2010. Automatic colorimetric calibration of human wounds. *BMC Med Imaging*, 10, pp. 1–12.

Wiemker, R., Dharaiya, E.D. & Bülow, T., 2012. Informatics in radiology: Hesse rendering for computer-aided visualization and analysis of anomalies at chest CT and breast MR imaging. *Radiographics*, pp. 289–304.

DICOM Calibration and GSDF

8

Key Points

The Human Visual System (HVS) perceives image intensities in a very nonlinear fashion. Barten's HVS model uses the concept of Just Noticeable Differences (JND) to capture the human vision LUT. DICOM calibration adopts Barten's model and applies it to undo the nonlinear effects of HVS.

8.1 Barten's Model

You might have heard about DICOM calibration a million times. But what is it doing, really?

A very neat thing: DICOM calibration compensates for the nonlinearities in our visual system. This is exactly what we discussed earlier: the human visual system has a very nonlinear response to the original pixel values. Can we correct this non-linearity with some smart choice of display lookup table? (Fig. 8.1).

It turns out that we can – if we know how our vision responds to the true pixel intensities. We already had a few hints of a solution when we talked about gamma correction, using $\gamma > 1$ to take advantage of our "night vision". This was a rather simple approximation, but fortunately HVS has been fascinating scientific minds long enough to have been studied to a good extent. Moreover, HVS has been *tabulated* just like any other display LUT. Among many HVS LUTs suggested by researchers, the DICOM standard picked Barten's model, shown in Fig. 8.2 (Barten 1992, 1999; Flynn 2012). As a result, this model has become particularly famous under the name of DICOM *Grayscale Display Function* (GSDF, Part 14 of DICOM standard).

It's worth understanding what this model actually describes. Barten was experimenting with a simple sinusoidal phantom (Fig. 8.2), changing the intensity of its central pattern to make it barely distinguishable from the background. The counts of those barely distinguishable shades were placed along the Fig. 8.2 horizontal axis; they were defined as *Just Noticeable Differences* (JNDs), the smallest detectable differences in shading that the average observer can perceive. The vertical axis shows the respective display luminance levels; the luminance of 500 cd/m², for

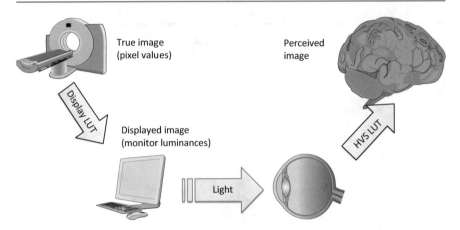

Fig. 8.1 Seeing images: from true to displayed and perceived

instance, allowed to distinguish 706 JNDs. By the very nature of the experiment we can associate JNDs with shades of gray; then the Barten model simply tells us how many distinct grayscales the HVS can detect at different monitor luminance levels.

▶ *Nota bene:* This is how Barten's model solves the eternal argument: how many shades of gray can a human being see? You may say 50 or 1,000, but it really depends on the luminance, as Barten's graph demonstrates; one cannot find a black cat in a dark room. See complete analysis in (Kimpe and Tuytschaever 2007). Also note that as luminance increases, Barten's curve becomes steeper, and our gain in JNDs becomes less and less significant (Fig. 8.2). Besides, you cannot increase luminance indefinitely: soon after 500 cd/m² it becomes too bright and tiring, and human eyes work less and less productively. Modern diagnostic monitors are usually in the 400–500 cd/m² luminance range, which translates into at most 706 simultaneous shades of visible gray.

But counting all noticeable differences is not all there is to GSDF; it's GSDF's curves that solve the HVS mystery. GSDF provides us with the perfect HVS LUT – the one we've been looking for to "straighten" the human visual nonlinearity. How? Consider two pixel values: $p_a = 706$, and its half, $p_b = 706/2 = 353$. If p_a is displayed with a bright dot of 500 cd/m², what brightness do we need for p_b so that our eyes perceive it as half of p_a? If your answer is $500/2 = 250$ cd/m², then think again, and revisit Fig. 8.2. You will see that the JND of 353 corresponds to some 37 cd/m², a significantly lower value! But it does make sense – remember, we can see better in the dark intensity range.

For practical imaging applications this means that the diagnostic display LUT, mapping the original pixel values into the monitor pixel luminances, has to be calibrated to display the value of 353 with 37 cd/m²; only then will our eyes – and our brains – perceive it as half as bright as the 706 pixel value. That is, calibrating computer monitors with GSDF LUT makes our perception *linear, proportional to the true pixel values.* This becomes extremely important for diagnostic image reading. For instance,

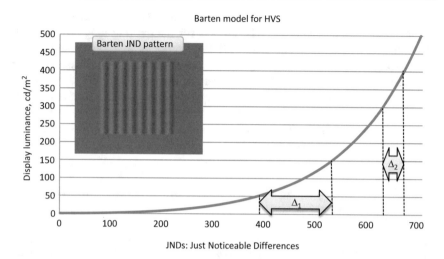

Fig. 8.2 Here it is, the famous Barten's JND curve, describing our ability to see different numbers of grayscale shades as a function of display luminance. The intensity of the sinusoidal pattern was gradually changed to make it barely visible over the background, and JNDs were counted at different luminance levels. Values of Δ_1 and Δ_2 show gains in JND produced by 100 cd/m² luminance increase at two different luminance levels. Note that as display luminance grows, we gain fewer and fewer JNDs

consider a CT image with two different tissues – one averaging 50 HU, and the other 100 HU. You really would like to perceive the second one as twice as bright as the first – then you would see the true tissue densities (HU values), and not what HVS transforms them into. Calibrating displays to GSDF LUT makes this happen.

▶ *Nota bene:* Although GSDF is commonly known as "DICOM calibration", there is really nothing "DICOM" about it. As you should see by now, it simply compensates for our intrinsically-nonlinear HVS. GSDF LUT makes our vision perceptually linear. Any other areas of human knowledge where this compensation matters –image compression and watermarking among them – can take advantage of GSDF (Wolfgang et al. 1999; Kutter and Winkler 2002)

To conclude: GSDF helps us see the real pixel values, and this makes diagnostic image interpretation less subjective. This is why DICOM calibration has become a routine maintenance procedure for PACS workstations, with calibration sensors often built into the monitor hardware. It's a slightly more challenging exercise for your home PC or smartphone, as they have no light sensors to measure their luminance output. Nevertheless, you can reasonably calibrate these devices using Barten's approach: looking at simple shading patterns and answering the questions of how many different shades you can see. And this is exactly how smartphone and "mobile" calibrations get the job done.[1]

---

[1] See http://www.barco.com/en/News/Press-releases/barco-launches-qa-and-calibration-tool-for-mobile-viewing-of-medical-images-on-the-ipad.aspx

If you are curious whether the GSDF concept can be explored any further, think about questions like "What LUT is the best for interpreting lung tumors?" The solution may be very different from GSDF (Uemura et al. 2006), pointing us to the organ-specific LUTS and totally different level of complexity. This essentially supersedes the basic W/L discussed at the very beginning of our LUT study; sophisticated organ-specific LUTs, at least in theory, can equip us with a better diagnostic view compared to simple W/L linear maps. Nonetheless, always keep in mind that any complexity leads to subjectivity and implementation bottlenecks. For now, let's appreciate the universality of GSDF, applicable to any image regardless of its content.

8.2   Bits Matter

> *chris k "It's not how many notes. It's how you play them."*
> *hezixiao "Well said. And it's not how many notes, it's how each one is written."*
> YouTube users on Mozart's Gran Partita

Our study of display LUTs would be completely theoretical if we forgot about the most important part: all digital images and display LUTs are *discrete*. This is what the T in LUT stands for – LUTs can hold only tabulated, finite sets of numbers. Moreover, these numbers can be stored only with finite computer precision, often rounded to the nearest integer. Anything below this precision will be truncated (*quantized*) to the nearest available match. This makes quantization error another important player in any LUT implementation, and it certainly affects our diagnostic viewing.

You don't need to be a computer scientist to figure this out, and here is how it works. Computers, our wonderful wired friends, store all information as binary numbers, the ranges of supported data values are usually measured in bits. As usual, N bits can be used to store 2^N possible discrete values. That's why, for example, the DICOM standard uses *bits stored, B_s,* to describe the "bit depth" of medical images: X-ray and CT images usually have $B_s = 12$ (meaning $2^{Bs} = 2^{12} = 4,096$ possible shades), X-rays may have B_s up to 16 ($2^{16} = 65,536$ possible shades).[2] Similarly, computer hardware (displays and graphics boards) are characterized by the maximum number of grayscale bits they can display, B_d. For conventional monitors, grayscale $B_d = 8$ (meaning up to $2^8 = 256$ different shades of gray). For advanced monitors used in radiology and other sciences, B_d can be as high as 12.

It's commonly assumed that image bit depth B_s has been set correctly to portray all required diagnostic details – this is why the DICOM standard prescribes optimal B_s values for different medical image types. Besides, once an image is acquired, we cannot improve its B_s, already carved in the granite of stored pixel values. And although keeping high B_s for DICOM data is certainly great, we cannot "see" images in DICOM files; we need them on a screen. That is, we need to match DICOM's B_s with a reasonable selection of the display's B_d values (Fig. 8.3).

---

[2] Part 3 of DICOM standard.

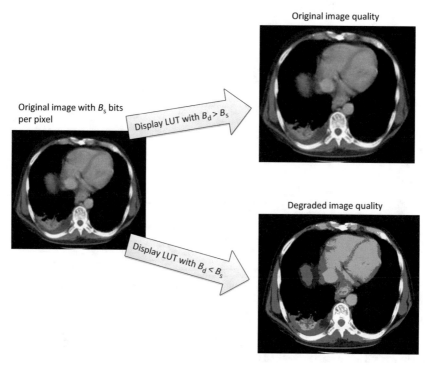

Fig. 8.3 When display LUT does not have enough intensity levels (B_d bits) to display all pixel values in the original image (B_s bits), several pixel values will be mapped into the same display value. This can manifest itself with lost image details and flattened intensities

What bit count would be sufficient to make our visual system happy? To find the answer, let's go back to Barten's model, where a typical and comfortable monitor brightness of 500 cd/m² gives us some 700 JNDs. Those can be packed into a 10-bit LUT: $B_d = 10$ provides $2^{10} = 1,024$ display shades. Problem solved?

Not at all! Have we forgotten that our intensity perception is completely non-linear? What it means in reality is that if we try to round JND curve numbers to their nearest finite-precision values, we get a pretty unpleasant result, shown in Fig. 8.4. Nonlinear JND will produce an extremely nonlinear quantization, where large ranges in the low intensities will be jammed into single quantized values. Required for computer LUT implementation, JND quantization will *downgrade* the quality of JND mapping, and as a result – the quality of our diagnostic image viewing.

Can this somehow be cured? Not really; computers play by their own rules, so we have to stay with the quantized LUT approach. Therefore, the only practical way to alleviate LUT roundoff errors is to lower the quantization step by tossing a few extra bits in B_d; for example, using $B_d = 11$ or $B_d = 12$ instead of the original $B_d = 10$. This will make final precision math in the quantized LUT a bit more precise, and quantization errors – smaller. This is exactly how medical hardware manufacturers end up with 11-bit radiological monitors.

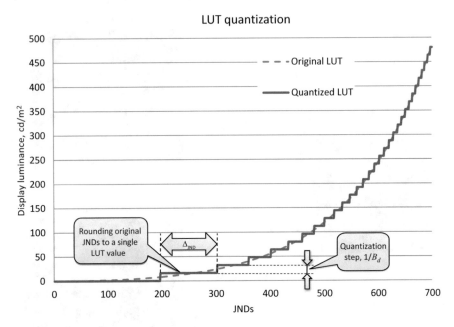

Fig. 8.4 GSDF LUT quantization: true (original) LUT values are rounded to discrete (quantized) luminances, supported by particular display hardware. See how large ranges of JNDs such as $\mathbf{\Delta}_{\mathrm{JND}}$ will be merged into a single quantized luminance, thus significantly degrading display quality. The only practical way to mitigate the negative effects of quantization is to use smaller quantization steps (higher number of available display luminances B_d)

But guess what? Simple "bit tossing" comes with a price tag of more expensive display hardware required to support more B_d bits. And as a result, the question of how many shades you would like to see turns into the question of how many grayscale shades you can *afford*. Going from the 8-bit consumer monitor to the advanced 11-bit LUT of professional displays may mean an order of magnitude price hike. Moreover, our dearly loved tablets and smartphones do not offer 11-bit displays, and won't any time soon. Therefore you should always end up weighing grayscale variety and radiologist satisfaction vs. hardware cost. Fortunately for your pockets and your patients, many studies indicate that most radiologists might even prefer 8-bit monitors as perceptually better (Bender et al. 2011) (Fig. 8.5).

The cost-value argument explains the imperishable popularity of our good old linear W/L transform. Seeing 1,024 shades of gray on a conventional 8-bit monitor is plain impossible – you can get 256 at best. But 1,024 original shades cover the entire image range, while what you need to see at any given time usually limits itself to a particular organ or tissue. If the human liver or brain has no more than some 100 shades, then you can easily W/L into them, making their finest details very distinct. This ability to "zoom" into selected intensity ranges efficiently counterweights the limitations of affordable display hardware. Ironic as it may sound, this turns W/L into our major cost-saving tool: you have to keep clicking on that W/L button to avoid buying expensive display hardware.

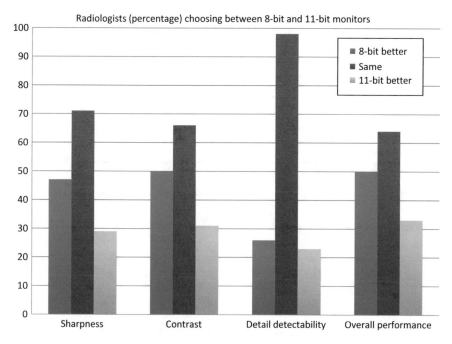

Fig. 8.5 Comparing 8-bit and 11-bit image display in Bender et al. study: most radiologists did not see any difference, and many favored 8-bit monitors as providing better image display

8.3 GSDF Math: How Curved Is the GSDF Curve?

It's worth spending a few more minutes to explore the shape of the GSDF curve.

Barten's GSDF LUT originated from his HVS model, tabulated for the first 1,023 JND values (from 1 to 1,023). You can find these GSDF LUT values in Part 14 of DICOM standard.[3] Figure 8.6 shows the resulting GSDF curve (in blue) – a larger view of the same curve that we had in Fig. 8.2 for the first 700 JNDs.

The same Part 14 of the DICOM standard provides us with a pretty impressive formula, that closely approximates the logarithm[4] of GSDF values as a function of JND level j:

$$\log_{10}(L) = \frac{a + c\ln(j) + r\ln^2(j) + g\ln^3(j) + m\ln^4(j)}{1 + b\ln(j) + d\ln^2(j) + f\ln^3(j) + h\ln^4(j) + k\ln^5(j)}, \tag{8.1}$$

where

$$a = -1.3011877; \quad b = -0.025840191; \quad c = 0.080242636;$$
$$d = -0.10320229; \quad r = 0.13646699; \quad f = 0.028745620;$$
$$g = -0.025468404; \quad h = -0.0031978977;$$
$$k = 0.00012992634; \quad m = 0.0013635334$$

---

[3] See current list of all DICOM parts at http://medical.nema.org/standard.html.

[4] As usual, $\log_{10}$ is the logarithm base 10, and $\ln = \log_e$ – the natural logarithm

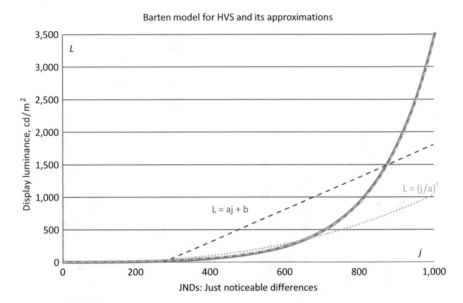

Fig. 8.6 Approximating Barten's GSDF

This formula offers a very good fit to the actual GSDF values (0.3 % relative error, 0.0003 standard deviation), therefore you can use it in any software or computation. However the sheer complexity of Eq. (8.1) sheds no light on the GSFD growth trend. At the same time, you can find a wealth of papers proposing GSFD approximations with linear, gamma, and other readily available hardware LUT. Maybe we can ditch expensive DICOM-calibration tools and calibrate our displays with a less demanding technique? For example, run DICOM calibration with a simple gamma-correction option available in nearly all monitor settings?

Let's examine our data a bit more closely. First, if you're thinking about using linear LUT to achieve DICOM calibration, look again at the straight line in Fig. 8.6. Pretty poor match, isn't it? Conclusion: computer monitors cannot be DICOM-calibrated with simple brightness/contrast adjustments; this is an obvious mathematical result, and it hardly needs any further investigation (Jervis and Brettle 2003).

Now look at the green curve in Fig. 8.6. This is the best GSDF approximation with a power function. Do you recognize this power equation? You should by now – this is our gamma correction. And if you want to use gamma to optimally tune your display into GSDF over the entire 700 JND range, your best bet would be $\gamma = 4$, as Table 8.1 suggests (which explains the use of similar gammas in many types of display hardware). As you can see, gamma LUT works far better than linear – in fact, if your display luminance is below 500 cd/m², gamma does a pretty good job. Yet it fails to keep up with the GSDF trend as display luminance increases.

Table 8.1 Approximations to GSDF LUT. Exponential approximation provides the lowest error, but gamma correction comes close in the 1–700 JND range (corresponding to up to 500 cd/m² luminance of conventional monitors)

Approximation type	Formula	JND range	Optimal coefficients minimizing maximum error	Maximum error (from GSDF)	Standard deviation (from GSDF)
Linear (contrast/brightness)	$L = aj + b$	1–1,023	$a = 3.907301$ $b = -1134.44$	1130.671	699.772
		1–700	$a = 0.683726$ $b = -295.669$	295.0356	69.13697
Power (gamma)	$L = (j/a)^\gamma$	1–1,023	$a = 247.5453$ $\gamma = 5.831963$	68.96223	38.26863
		1–700	$a = 154.3977$ $\boldsymbol{\gamma = 4.072386}$	8.673658	5.329051
Exponential, $exp(x) = e^x$	$L = ae^{j/b} + c$	1–1,023	$a = 4.808426$ $b = 152.1229$ $c = 3.275661$	11.44335	7.736478
		1–700	$a = 3.833774$ $b = 145.317$ $c = 3.277577$	7.09767	4.80447

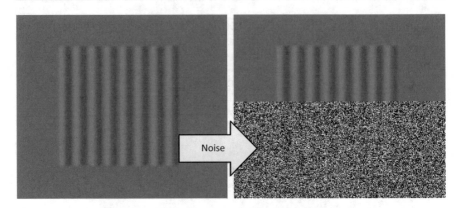

Fig. 8.7 Noise can significantly reduce our ability to differentiate between image shades and patterns. After we added some Gaussian noise to the bottom half of the Barten image, it essentially masked the JND shading pattern, clearly visible before

If GSDF grows faster than the power function, then the next thing that comes to mind is the exponent. I did a little analysis, and found the following exponential approximation to GSDF (Table 8.1):

$$L_E(j) = ae^{j/b} + c \tag{8.2}$$

This curve is shown in Fig. 8.6 with a yellow dashed line – as you can see, it looks nearly indistinguishable from the true GSDF curve.[5] The fact that our visual system perceives grayscale shades with almost exponential LUT explains why linear and power functions cannot fit the alluring GSDF growth.[6] This also explains why a slight increase in the desired count of JNDs can require enormous increases in luminance.

Finally, for the pure math aficionados, I can offer an even better GSDF approximation:

$$L_{ES}(j) = ae^{j/b} + c + d\sin(\omega j), \tag{8.3}$$

where

$$a = 5.1630823717991; \quad b = 153.730653509978;$$
$$c = -9.83587722126755,$$
$$\omega = -0.0393; \quad d = -9.99191252364592$$

with maximum error of 0.94 cd/m². It has the same exponential trend, with a bounded sine wave added to achieve better approximation in the medium JND range.

Formulas are fun, and can be exercised indefinitely, but make no mistake: our HVS is much more complex than any of its formal models. Your perception of shades and details depends on lighting, distance, background, image artifacts (such as noise, Fig. 8.7), your fatigue and many other factors – possibly including your diet and the

---

[5] For small j, $L_E(j)$ can have negative values, so take the absolute value.

[6] See Weber-Fechner law on Wikipedia.

movie you watched yesterday. Consider ambient lightning, ignored by GSDF: it's dark in the radiology reading rooms, but it's brightly lit in the referring physicians' offices; this discrepancy can often result in completely different perception of the same image. Mach bands in Fig. III.1 are another example – even on the most calibrated monitor you will still "see" grayscale deviations that simply do not exist.

Nevertheless, knowing the basics of GSDF curvature provides us with a very reliable approach to objective diagnostic viewing. The rest, my dear reader – finally! –depends on your professional training.

8.4 Self-check

8.4.1 Questions

1. If HVS needs at most 11-bit LUT, why does DICOM support up to 16-bit grayscale images?
2. What is the maximum number of grayscales you might be able to see on your smartphone?
3. Name all HVS-related "obstacles" between the original image data and your interpretation of it.

8.4.2 Answers

1. Well, did I say that HVS is the ultimate diagnostic tool? Once again, think about CAD – when computers analyze pixel values, they can surely "perceive" the smallest numerical differences, and take advantage of the entire 16-bit range (or more). The goal of DICOM is not to match the subjective HVS standards; instead, it is to capture the original data as accurately as possible. This is when higher precision counts.
2. Check the technical specs for your favorite gadget, and map its display brightness onto our JND curve – then you will see how many JNDs to expect. Note that the display still needs optimal GSDF calibration, and the actual display brightness may not be set up to 100 %. But whatever JND count you get, compare it with the grayscale resolution you expect to see in your images. For instance, if you need to work with intensity ranges some 300 or 400 units wide, do you have enough JNDs to see them?
3. We discussed at least the following ones:
   (a) Our nonlinear perception of pixel intensities. That's why we need GSDF LUT (Barten's curve) to undo it.
   (b) LUT quantization. When Barten's function is used in a computer finite-precision LUT, we lose accuracy because of quantization.
   (c) Hardware. Your display hardware needs to be chosen to match the bit depth of your quantized LUT.

References

Barten, P.G., 1992. Physical model for the Contrast Sensitivity of the human eye. San Jose, CA, SPIE, pp. 57–72.

Barten, P.G., 1999. Contrast Sensitivity of the Human Eye and Its Effects on Image Quality. s.l.:SPIE.

Bender, S. et al., 2011. 8-bit or 11-bit monochrome displays–which image is preferred by the radiologist?. *Eur Radiol,* pp. 1088–1096.

Flynn, M., 2012. DICOM Basics Pertaining to Displays. In: *Displays.* s.l.:SIIM, pp. Online: http://siimcenter.org/books/displays/chapter-3-dicom-basics-pertaining-displays.

Jervis, S.E. and Brettle, D.S., 2003. A practical approach to soft-copy display consistency for PC-based review workstations. *British Journal of Radiology,* pp. 648–652.

Kimpe, T. and Tuytschaever, T., 2007. Increasing the number of gray shades in medical display systems–how much is enough? *Journal of Digital Imaging,* pp. 422–432.

Kutter, M. & Winkler, S., 2002. A vision-based masking model for spread-spectrum image watermarking. *IEEE Transactions on Image Processing,* pp. 16–25.

Uemura, M. et al., 2006. Psychophysical evaluation of calibration curve for diagnostic LCD monitor. *Radiat Med,* pp. 653–658.

Wolfgang, R.B., Podilchuk, C.I. and Delp, E.J., 1999. Perceptual watermarks for digital images and video. *Proceedings of the IEEE,* pp. 1108–1126.

Conclusion

9

Imagine one of those rare days, my sophisticated reader, when you do not need to rush in the morning; and not even for the rest of the day. So you wake up, get your fresh latte, slide into a comfortable chair, close your eyelids and think about very complex things. Occasionally, you make little philosophical discoveries, and you realize that many complex things are related, often spawning from the same roots. Suddenly and finally, it all starts making sense. You are sitting in your cave, watching the dancing shadows on the walls, which are nothing but the reflections from a single fire. Sound familiar?

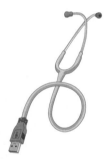

If you had such a moment reading this book, it would make me happy, and my goal – fulfilled.

Printed in the United States
By Bookmasters